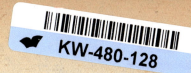

# Heart Attacks Understood

Dr Ian Anderson, MB, BS, LRCP, MRCS, qualified at Guy's Hospital, London, in 1964. From 1971 to 1976 he ran the Cardiac Rehabilitation Unit at the Kent and Sussex Hospital, and in 1976 was awarded the Upjohn Travelling Fellowship for Cardiac Rehabilitation. He is an Honorary Research Fellow in Exercise Testing at St Mary's Hospital, London, and has his own cardiac rehabilitation and exercise testing unit in Harley Street.

Dr Ian Anderson

# Heart Attacks Understood

illustrated by Chris Evans

**Pan Books** in association with Macmillan

## Acknowledgement

I should like to thank Dr Peter Hewlett Kidner, MA, MB, BS, FRCP, Consultant Physician and Cardiologist at St Mary's Hospital, Paddington, for his help and encouragement over the years and particularly for reading the proofs of this book.

First published 1980 by Macmillan London Ltd
This edition published 1981 by Pan Books Ltd,
Cavaye Place, London SW10 9PG
in association with Macmillan London Ltd
© Dr Ian Anderson 1980
ISBN 0 330 26318 8
Printed and bound in Great Britain by
Richard Clay (The Chaucer Press) Ltd, Bungay, Suffolk

# Contents

# Introduction

'Have you heard about poor old Smithy? He hadn't been feeling too good lately – well, you know there's been all that trouble over the half-yearly accounts – he suddenly went ashen last week. Terrible pains in his chest and throat – whipped off in an ambulance to hospital – heart attack!' This is an all too familiar account nowadays – and the people talking will probably first feel sorry for John Smith, then relieved that they are not in his shoes; they will send him a get-well card and go on to the latest cricket scores, and there, for them, the matter ends – or does it?

If we look at the overall pattern of the incidence of heart attacks, we will see that either of John Smith's two colleagues could well be the next to be 'whipped off in an ambulance'. Infectious diseases such as tuberculosis, diphtheria and cholera used to be the prime killers, but heart attacks are now the most common cause of death in any country rich enough to publish statistics. In Europe alone, about a million people a year die as a result of a heart attack – a number exceeding the records established for the Great Plague. If you imagine Wembley on Cup Final Day, then add half as many people again – *that* is the number of people in Britain who die from heart attacks every year.

# Death rates from coronary disease in different countries, per 100,000 population, aged 55-64 years

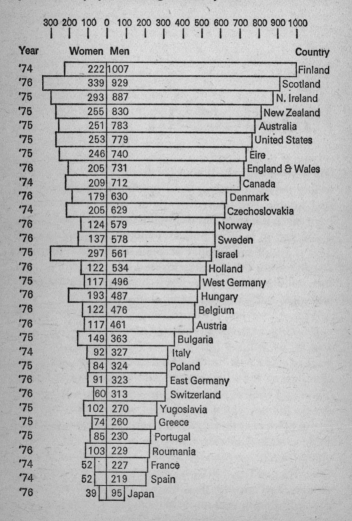

| Year | Women | Men | Country |
|------|-------|-----|---------|
| '74 | 222 | 1007 | Finland |
| '76 | 339 | 929 | Scotland |
| '75 | 293 | 887 | N. Ireland |
| '75 | 255 | 830 | New Zealand |
| '75 | 251 | 783 | Australia |
| '75 | 253 | 779 | United States |
| '75 | 246 | 740 | Eire |
| '76 | 205 | 731 | England & Wales |
| '74 | 209 | 712 | Canada |
| '76 | 179 | 630 | Denmark |
| '74 | 205 | 629 | Czechoslovakia |
| '76 | 124 | 579 | Norway |
| '76 | 137 | 578 | Sweden |
| '75 | 297 | 561 | Israel |
| '76 | 122 | 534 | Holland |
| '75 | 117 | 496 | West Germany |
| '76 | 193 | 487 | Hungary |
| '76 | 122 | 476 | Belgium |
| '76 | 117 | 461 | Austria |
| '75 | 149 | 363 | Bulgaria |
| '74 | 92 | 327 | Italy |
| '75 | 84 | 324 | Poland |
| '76 | 91 | 323 | East Germany |
| '76 | 60 | 313 | Switzerland |
| '75 | 102 | 270 | Yugoslavia |
| '75 | 74 | 260 | Greece |
| '75 | 85 | 230 | Portugal |
| '76 | 103 | 229 | Roumania |
| '74 | 52 | 227 | France |
| '74 | 52 | 219 | Spain |
| '76 | 39 | 95 | Japan |

Exactly how many heart attacks there are annually in Britain is not known, for they are not notifiable – unlike measles, for example, which requires notification to a central statistical body. In England the incidence has increased fourfold in thirty years, in Scotland even more, and although in other countries the increase began at different times, the current trend is the same in all. These figures continue to rise, and according to the World Health Organization heart disease has reached epidemic proportions. It is a salutary thought that if all forms of cancer were made totally preventable, the average life expectancy of a man would increase by 2.6 years and that of a woman by 2.7 years, while if all forms of heart disease were preventable, a man's average life expectancy would increase by 7 years, a woman's by 9 years.

A mass of information has been accumulated about the causes of heart attacks, treatment of the attack and problems resulting from it, and, more recently, about those who survive an attack, but John Smith and his colleagues – the average men in the street – know very little about it, and probably, since most of us have a bit of the ostrich in us, don't want to know. But nothing breeds fear like ignorance, and the purpose of this book is to try and explain the heart, how it works and how it can be abused, and what happens when a heart attack occurs; to show why there are specialized units in hospitals to deal with the crisis and why these should be reassuring and not terrifying to the patient and his family; and to give some idea of what can be expected after a heart attack – especially to explode the myth that 'heart attacks must rest'. It is unlikely that, having read this book, you will become a heart specialist or an authority on coronary heart disease, but I hope that the destructive fear of the unknown and much of the mystique surrounding this disease will be replaced by understanding and a reassuring basic knowledge. Some of the information, like the chapter on the anatomy of the heart, its valves and blood supply, may seem unnecessarily technical, but in order to understand what can go wrong you need to know how the heart works normally.

At the beginning of this introduction I gave some gloomy facts about death rates. But the weight of evidence is that it is possible to reduce the chance of becoming one of these statistics – hence the chapter on the 'risk factors', smoking, overweight, stress and so on, and how you can avoid these. One eminent cardiologist feels so strongly about potential preventive action that he considers a heart attack to be 'a self-inflicted disease', which may be overstating the case but makes the point.

Wherever possible I have tried to avoid using statistics, since so much work on heart disease is going on all over the world, and often the findings and observations are in conflict – which is the way of all research and advances in medicine. I have used the least controversial statistics, and the conclusions you read in this book are those which are now most generally accepted in the medical profession. It has also proved impossible to avoid using some unfamiliar terminology, and explanations of these terms may be found in the Glossary on page 148.

# 1 How the Heart Works

Why you have a heart attack and what happens during one can only be understood when you have some knowledge of the normal heart and how it works.

## The heart

The heart itself is a hollow muscular organ, almost conical in shape, with the base at the top and the apex pointing downwards. It weighs from 225 grams to 350 grams in men, slightly less in women. Its size is related to the size of the body: it is usually roughly the same size as the clenched fist of the subject. The position of the heart varies considerably depending on the shape of the chest and the height of the diaphragm, a muscular umbrella which separates the chest cavity from the abdominal cavity. The apex of the heart is situated between the 5th and 6th ribs on the left side of the chest, on a line downwards from the middle of the collar bone; the right side of the heart is just to the right of the breastbone.

The heart is divided into two sides separated by a thin wall, the *septum*; each side has two chambers: the top, thin-walled collecting area called the *atrium*, which leads into

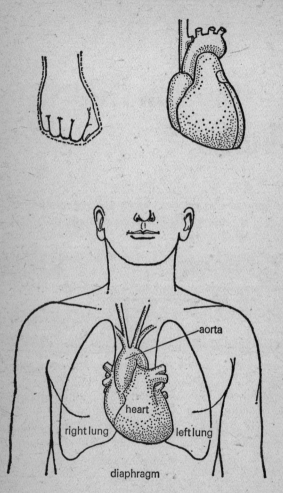

*The size of a person's heart compares roughly with the size of his clenched fist. The lower diagram shows the position of the heart in relation to the lungs. The base of the heart is at the top, the apex at the bottom on the left side of the chest.*

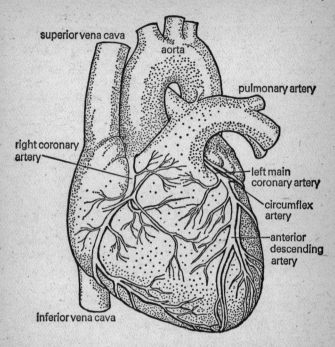

*The heart's blood supply. The right and left coronary arteries leave the aorta, the left dividing into the anterior descending and circumflex arteries.*

the bottom, thick, muscular-walled pumping unit called the *ventricle*.

The heart is the central powerhouse of the entire body circulation. Blood comes in on one side and is pumped out on the other – refuelled with oxygen. The expulsion of the waste, carbon dioxide, and collection of oxygen takes place in the lungs, so two balanced circulations are needed: one going all round the body with blood rich in vital oxygen, and the other going through the lungs getting rid of the waste carbon dioxide and picking up the oxygen.

The blood coming from round the body back to the heart through the veins, enters the right atrium through two large vessels – the *superior vena cava,* bringing blood down from the head and entering the roof, and the *inferior vena cava,* bringing blood up from the rest of the body and entering the back wall. The floor of the right atrium is a valve – the *tricuspid valve* – through which the blood passes to enter the right ventricle.

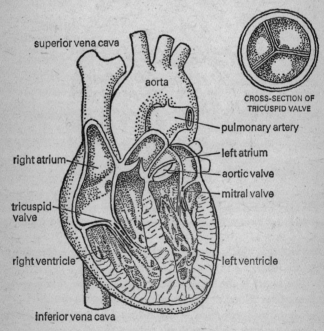

superior vena cava

aorta

CROSS-SECTION OF
TRICUSPID VALVE

pulmonary artery

right atrium

left atrium

aortic valve

mitral valve

tricuspid
valve

right ventricle

left ventricle

inferior vena cava

*The valvular system of the heart. Deoxygenated blood collects in the right atrium and passes through the tricuspid valve into the right ventricle and then to the lungs. After oxygenation the blood returns to the left atrium and passes into the large muscular left ventricle through the mitral valve, and then round the body via the aortic valve.*

The right ventricle is a muscular chamber; the inside walls are irregular due to muscular columns, some of which have small tendon-like cords stretching from the wall itself to the valve edges and enabling the valve to open and shut. The chamber is like a bent tube, the main part of which collects blood from the atrium through the tricuspid valve, and the smaller end leads into the *pulmonary artery*, the big vessel taking blood to the lungs for refuelling. The opening of the pulmonary artery is guarded by another valve with three cusps – each cusp is a flap of skin-like tissue and at the centre of each free edge is a small lump or nodule, which combines with the other two to ensure a perfect closure of the valve by filling the gap which would occur at the meeting of the three flaps. So the blood returning to the central pump for refuelling arrives at the collecting station, the right atrium, through the two huge veins called the vena cavae. It passes through a valve into the right ventricle which contracts, and because of the arrangement of the valves, can only go one way – through another valve into the pulmonary artery and to the lungs.

The pulmonary artery divides into two branches – one to each lung – and then sub-divides into a fine network of blood vessels which surround the tiny air sacs of the lungs. As the blood flows through the lungs it gives up the carbon dioxide and absorbs the oxygen, then returns to the left side of the heart through the pulmonary veins. In case you are already confused by the difference between arteries and veins, arteries are the thick, muscular-walled blood vessels taking blood *away* from the heart; veins are the thin-walled vessels bringing blood *back* to the heart. Generally arteries carry oxygenated blood, veins deoxygenated – the only exception being the pulmonary circulation. The four pulmonary veins enter the heart through the back wall of the left atrium, which is slightly smaller than the right. The pulmonary veins do not have valves, but the floor of the left atrium is the *mitral valve*, formed in this case of two cusps, one much larger than the other. The mitral valve leads into the largest and most muscular chamber of the heart – the left ventricle. From here the blood is pumped around the whole body, so although the left ventricle is similar in formation to the right, having the same small cords from the inner wall to the valve, it has to be more powerful, and its muscular wall is therefore two and a half to three times thicker. Out of the left ventricle, the blood is pumped into the huge main artery of the body – the *aorta* – again through a valve. The *aortic valve* is similar to the valve in the pulmonary artery, but behind each cusp the valve is pouched out to form a small pocket, called the *sinus of Valsalva*.

If, understandably, you have by now forgotten the beginning of this journey, let us summarize it once again. Blood for refuelling enters the right side of the heart – is collected in the right atrium – passes into the right ventricle – to the pulmonary arteries – to the lungs, where carbon dioxide is given up and oxygen absorbed – returns to the left side of the heart in the pulmonary vein – to the left atrium – into the left ventricle and out into the body circulation through the aorta. Thus there are two circuits from the same pump, each circuit being separated in the heart by the thin wall called the septum.

Incidentally, this wall sometimes has a congenital defect of a hole between the atria or the ventricles which entirely upsets the efficiency of the two circuits, as the deoxygenated blood gets mixed with the oxygenated blood. Babies born with this defect – known as 'blue babies' – consequently suffer from too little oxygen in the circulating blood, though fortunately the holes can now be repaired by surgery – the hole in the heart operation.

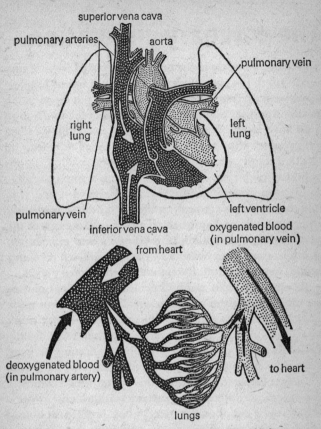

superior vena cava

pulmonary arteries — aorta

pulmonary vein

right lung

left lung

pulmonary vein

left ventricle

inferior vena cava

oxygenated blood (in pulmonary vein)

from heart

deoxygenated blood (in pulmonary artery)

to heart

lungs

*A simplified diagram (top) showing the direction of the blood circulation (the heart and lungs are not to scale). Deoxygenated blood collects in the right side of the heart and is then pumped via the pulmonary arteries to the lungs. After oxygenation the blood returns in the pulmonary veins to the left ventricle of the heart, and then leaves via the aorta for circulation around the body. The lower diagram shows how the large vessels carrying deoxygenated blood from the heart break down to a very fine network within the lungs, where the gaseous exchange takes place before the blood returns to the heart.*

# The coronary circulation

Almost every muscle in the body can be rested when it gets tired. Not so the poor old heart muscle – it has to keep at it, non-stop, irrespective of the demands put upon it. It usually manages extremely well, but in order to do so it must have an efficient fuel supply of its own. This is called the coronary circulation, and it is problems or defects in this that result in coronary artery disease.

Behind each cusp of the aortic valve is a small pocket – called, you remember, the sinus of Valsalva – and it is from here that the coronary arteries arise. So, immediately after the aorta, and just behind the skin flap cusps of the aortic valve, is the origin of the heart's own circulation, which has two main branches – the right and left coronary artery, stemming from the right and left coronary sinus.

In order to avoid using difficult and technical names, we can visualize the coronary circulation as a road map. Clearly visible at a glance are the motorways – huge trunk roads carrying vast amounts of traffic. Then there are the A roads, major carriageways linking important or large areas; the B roads, smaller but still important in linking the major roads to the lanes – tiny routes which complete the complicated network of carriageways which, provided the system is not abused or overloaded, is quite capable of dealing with the traffic load. Accidents, however, can happen and even the huge motorways will become blocked if there is a multiple pile-up; this analogy, related to the coronary circulation, will show the mechanism of coronary artery disease and its effects.

The motorways are the right and left coronary arteries, arising from the aorta. The left artery is the main motorway, varying in length from a few millimetres to a few centimetres; it divides into two branches – themselves of sufficient size and importance to be considered motorways also – the *anterior descending* going downwards, the *circumflex* branching off at right angles and continuing around the heart.

As the anterior descending artery goes down between the two ventricles it gives off branches – A roads. The first of these joins up with the right coronary artery to form a ring; the others, one, two or three, branch off, making A

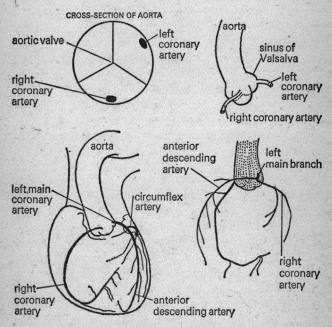

*Coronary artery circulation. The two main coronary arteries arise directly from the aorta. The left main branch divides into two large arteries, the anterior descending and the circumflex, which supply the front and left side of the heart. The right coronary artery passes to the back of the heart.*

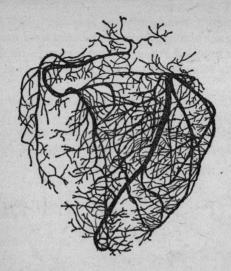

*The complete circulation of the heart. Each of the major vessels has several tributaries which form an intricate pattern of intercommunicating arteries.*

roads to supply the heart muscle wall. The motorway itself travels right down to the apex of the heart, then turns upwards for a short distance to the back of the heart, between the ventricles.

The second branch of the left main motorway, the circumflex, goes off around the heart between the atrium and the ventricle, giving off several smaller branches on the way, and continues as a major A road down across the ventricle to the apex. In 45 per cent of hearts examined, this artery gives off a branch to supply the area of the heart which controls the heart beat and rhythm – the pacemaker, which is a nerve centre controlled both by the brain and by chemicals circulating in the blood (not to be confused with the artificial pacemaker, see page 68).

The other main motorway leaving the aorta is the right coronary artery. This goes round the heart between the right atrium and ventricle, the A roads continuing to the apex of the right ventricle and down at the back of the heart, giving off branches all the way which eventually join up with the branches of the left artery; some of these branches go into the septum and – in the other 55 per cent – one goes to the pacemaking area.

The pacemaker – the heart's 'electrical system' – is a highly sensitive series of nerve bundles situated in the wall of the right atrium, running down the upper part between the ventricles and then dividing to form two bundles, one

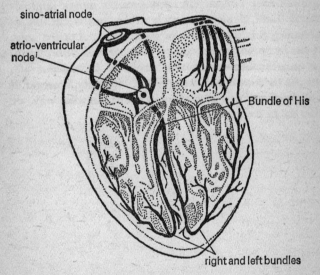

*The electrical system of the heart. The electrical impulse starts in the sino-atrial node and stimulates the atria to contract. The atrioventricular node is then stimulated and the current passes via the Bundle of His to the right and left bundles, causing the ventricles to contract.*

supplying each ventricle. In situations of fear or excitement the brain will stimulate these nerves, causing the heart to increase in rate and power so that the body is ready to cope with the demand. The blood supply for this system comes directly from the coronary artery branches, so any disease or disturbance of these vessels may well upset the regulation of heart rhythm.

The action of the heart is beautifully co-ordinated, an efficient pumping mechanism with valves opening and closing, blood flowing, and muscles contracting and relaxing at an average rate of 70 beats a minute in a healthy person under normal circumstances. It moves approximately 75ml of blood at each stroke, but is capable of increasing this volume five or six times when called upon by the brain, in an emergency. Starting long before birth, the heart continues beating regularly throughout life. Despite its exceptional strength and versatility, however, it is all too frequently abused by its owner. In what way, we shall see in the next chapter.

# 2 Risk Factors in Coronary Heart Disease

*Patient:* 'I've been reading about heart disease, Doctor. Now, if I give up smoking, drinking, gourmet eating and the high-pressure jetsetting job that I enjoy so much, would you guarantee that I won't have a heart attack and that I'll live longer?'

*Doctor:* 'No, no one can give you a guarantee that you won't have a heart attack, but give that lot up and however long you live, it will certainly seem a long time.'

## What is atherosclerosis?

Hardening of the arteries – known as atherosclerosis – is the result of a long-term process in which the vessel walls become lined with fatty tissue; it is the dominant cause of coronary artery disease. Atherosclerosis is not a natural part of growing older. Its origins are in infancy and childhood, and are accelerated in adolescence; the complications begin to appear in the middle or late years. It is now the most common single disease in the Western world.

In atherosclerosis the larger arteries are affected by two conditions, varying in degree: *plaques*, which are deposits in the lining of the arteries filled with fats (lipids), and *fibrosis*, loss of elasticity in the middle layer of the artery wall. Some people remain completely free of both conditions, but most adults have gone at least some way along the line and there is little harm done unless something like 50 per cent of an artery has been blocked, at which point it will probably be manifested clinically. The significance of the blockage is dependent upon the artery involved, particularly so if the artery is in the heart, when it is the cause of the massive problem of coronary heart disease.

Although the accumulating of fatty deposits begins in youth, it does not usually affect the coronary arteries – those supplying the heart muscle – until the third decade; the process continues and becomes more widespread throughout the body, although it is not until the fifth decade that the vessels to the brain are grossly affected. The deposits in the heart are laid down at the start of the heart's circulation, where the arteries are still in the surrounding fat and where the vessels divide within the heart wall at the junction of the two 'roads'. Exactly how these plaques develop is not quite clear, but small fatty streaks are often seen in areas of wear and tear in the lining of the artery, and these streaks develop into plaques. (See hypertension and raised blood cholesterol, pages 23 and 26.)

# The risks

There is little doubt that atherosclerosis is an example of a disease process to which many factors contribute; what *is* in question is just how much significance each of these factors has individually. There is no point in entering into a controversy about the order of significance of these risk factors, for it is more than likely that if you were to ask half

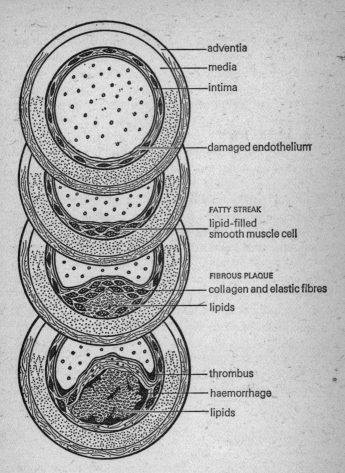

- adventia
- media
- intima
- damaged endothelium

**FATTY STREAK**
- lipid-filled smooth muscle cell

**FIBROUS PLAQUE**
- collagen and elastic fibres
- lipids

- thrombus
- haemorrhage
- lipids

*Hardening of the arteries. The process begins with damage to the lining of the blood vessel (the endothelium); the smooth muscle cells then increase and lipids accumulate. Collagen and elastic fibres develop, forming a fibrous plaque which protrudes into the blood vessel. Further tissue destruction and calcification with haemorrhage is the final advanced stage.*

a dozen doctors, you would get six different answers. Of course, there is always the enthusiast who believes that one thing is vastly more important than another: 'Avoid all fat', 'Avoid all stress', etc. In this chapter we will examine those factors which have been incriminated as significant and which are accepted with the least controversy.

## Family history

This is probably one of the most difficult yet most interesting factors to evaluate, as there are so many variables such as acquired patterns of diet and behaviour. But statistics do seem to show that there is a significantly greater risk for children of parents who have had premature evidence of atherosclerosis, i.e. if the father at less than 55 years old or the mother at less than 65 years has had a heart attack, then the child appears to have about seven times as high a chance of the disease as the general population; if the parents succumb at a later age, then the child's risk drops to about twice that of the general population. Other risk factors linked with heredity are discussed under individual headings.

It is worth noting, to reassure those whose parents have suffered a heart attack at an early age and who, in the light of these comments, might now consider themselves as 'marked men', that there is an enormous variability from one race or culture to another. Finland has the highest recorded incidence of heart disease in the world but in Sweden – close neighbour – it is only about 20 per cent as great; the United States is not far behind Finland but Japan has a very low incidence, yet when the Japanese emigrate to California, within two or three generations their rate reaches that of other Americans. So it may be that habit and environment accelerate atherosclerosis as much as purely genetic or hereditary predisposition.

# Smoking

Death from heart attack, particularly sudden death, is four times higher in smokers than non-smokers. People give numerous reasons for smoking: 'It gives me something to do with my hands', 'If I don't smoke, I put on weight', 'I only smoke if I'm bored', 'It helps me to concentrate' – none of which seems to justify furring up one's coronary arteries, sooting up one's lungs or playing Russian roulette between heart and lung disease.

Cigarette smoking involves the inhalation of poisonous tars and highly potent cancer-producing agents; if the habit is long established there is of course permanent, irreparable damage to the lungs. This may be in the form of cancer (cancer of the lung being a particularly lethal variety), or in the form of chronic bronchitis and emphysema, a condition in which the small air sacs in the lungs over-expand and secretions within the lung increase; this causes more coughing and the vicious circle goes on. All this is bad enough, but nicotine also has a direct action on the heart circulation. It increases the heart rate at rest as well as the consumption of oxygen by the heart muscle, with a corresponding constriction of the blood vessels; it also has an effect on the clotting mechanism and fat metabolism.

Cigarette smoke contains carbon monoxide – the gas used by suicides who stay in a locked garage with the car engine running – and it dissolves much more easily in the blood than oxygen does, in fact it latches itself on to the haemoglobin, the part of the blood carrying the oxygen, thus creating a blocking effect. Of course it takes longer to die through this mechanism by smoking cigarettes than by sitting in a garage with the car engine running, but the end result is the same.

If the heart circulation is already restricted by a mechanical blockage such as a plaque and you add the problem of blood partially poisoned by carbon monoxide, this alone can precipitate the symptoms of angina. (Angina is dealt with in detail in Chapter 3. It is sufficient to say that it is a symptom of heart disease – characteristically pain in the chest – which is brought on by activity, emotion or possibly food, and relieved by rest; it is caused by insufficient oxygen being supplied to the heart muscle.) For the sceptic I have a highly revealing procedure: I sit him down in front of the monitor (see page 123), give him a cigarette and let him watch the changes in his own heart-beat; several patients have given up smoking immediately.

It is all very well for a doctor to say to a patient 'You must give up smoking'. Nobody disputes the sanity of this advice, but it is a very difficult habit – if not addiction – to break. There is no easy way other than the will to succeed; but it does seem a pity that so often the motivation to stop is provided only by a heart attack. Almost without exception an increase in weight will be an immediate result of giving up smoking – no doubt eating replaces the oral gratification of the cigarette – but if this helps to break the habit, it is preferable in the short term to smoking. There is really no point in cutting down or rationing cigarettes, for as soon as a situation arises which can be used as an excuse for a smoke, the ration will go by the board and consumption will be back to the original figure.

Opinion varies about changing to a pipe or cigars. Some figures seem to show that these carry only 25 per cent of the risk involved, but the addicted tobacco smoker will inhale anyway and this will have a similar end result. So the only advice can be to give it up completely and, like the alcoholic, never take the odd one – before very long it will be the odd twenty.

# Raised blood pressure (hypertension)

In simple mechanical terms the heart is a pump, and as such is pushing fluid around a network of tubing. As with any pump, a certain pressure is required to keep the fluid moving. When you are watering the garden it is no use if the water is trickling out of the hose or, at the other end of the scale, coming out in a long, powerful jet; to do the job properly the pressure must be just right – too low and it's ineffective, too high and the rose gets blown off. As with the hose-pipe, the blood circulation has an optimum ideal pressure, and this varies with activity: the greater the demand the higher the pressure. If the resulting blood pressure is too high there is a definite increase in heart disease and other problems.

The blood pressure is measured using an instrument called a sphygmomanometer. An inflatable cuff attached to a column of mercury is placed around the upper arm. The cuff is inflated until the pulse at the elbow can no longer be felt; with the stethoscope placed over the artery, the cuff is slowly deflated, releasing the blood flow which will be heard through the stethoscope. The first sound is the upper reading – the systolic pressure; as the cuff is further deflated the noise of the blood flow gets louder then suddenly fades away, and at this point is the lower reading – the diastolic pressure. The textbook norm at rest for these figures is 120/80mmHg (millimetres of mercury). The figures vary with age and can be affected by other stimuli, such as exercise, emotion, fear, sex and stress. If the resting blood pressure is higher than normal the person is said to be suffering from *hypertension*, i.e. high blood pressure. This may show in a variety of symptoms like headaches, dizziness and palpitations, but very often the individual is completely unaware of the situation and it

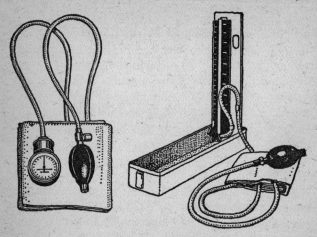

*Sphygmomanometers. Two types are in common use, the mercury (right) and the aneroid. Both have an inflatable cuff with a release valve; the blood pressure is read either as a column of mercury or directly on the dial.*

may only be discovered at a routine medical examination.

Hypertension is without doubt a highly potent risk factor in coronary heart disease, for which often no cause can be found. Although not often curable it can now be controlled by drugs. There is some disagreement in the medical profession about the level of blood pressure which may be called hypertensive, but it would seem that the 'ideal' blood pressure is not the 'normal' blood pressure, and there is a definite reduction in atherosclerosis in people with subnormal rather than so-called normal blood pressure. Low levels of hypertension have been found to increase atherosclerosis, threefold in men between 40 and 59 years old and sixfold in women of the same age. It is by no means a rare condition; about 15–20 per cent of a random population may be expected to show these levels, but few deaths are attributed to hypertension directly. Its complications in accelerating blood vessel disease in the heart and brain, however, underline it as a strong risk factor.

Raised blood pressure is thought to cause local areas of damage in the blood vessel wall and changes in the fat breakdown process which leads to the formation of the plaques characteristic of atherosclerosis. The combination of raised blood pressure, raised fat content in the blood and cigarette smoking seems to cause a particularly rapid progress of the disease.

## Obesity

If a car runs out of petrol it requires more fuel; if too much fuel is put in the tank, it overflows; if too much fuel reaches the pistons the engine will 'run rough'. If too much fuel, in the shape of food, is taken in the surplus tends to be laid down as fat, causing overweight which makes movement more difficult and the body less efficient. The body has a basic fuel requirement for everyday living. This varies from person to person, and in addition the energy expenditure will vary enormously according to your occupation. If your basic requirement is consistently exceeded, obesity will result, usually bringing with it a great variety of medical problems. People think it dangerous to overload an elevator by twice the recommended weight, but give little thought to the problems they create by overloading the one frame they have been given. Obesity not only causes problems affecting the artery walls and the heart muscle, it also puts long-term mechanical pressures on joints, producing painful backaches and arthritic conditions, particularly in the weight-bearing joints. Gall bladder and kidney conditions are just two of those directly related to obesity.

Clearly there are some elements of diet which are more closely related to heart disease than others, and the problem of animal fat is discussed below. Insurance companies – hardly charitable organizations – are only too well aware of the fact that being overweight carries a risk of early death, and increase their life assurance premiums accordingly. Their statistics show that people who are 20 per cent overweight – according to the ideal height/weight ratio, see chart on page 136 – have a higher death rate than those of standard risk; even 5kg overweight appears to carry a greater risk than smoking 25 cigarettes a day.

How does one lose weight? The first major step is to lose any complacency about obesity and have a genuine desire to reduce; once the motivation is achieved, the battle is half won. Basically the fuel has to be reduced, and the advice 'Eat what you usually eat but only eat half of it' is very sound. There are a hundred and one different diets and some will suit some people (there is a diet sheet and a calorie chart on pages 137 and 140), but the main ingredient of any one of them is the desire to succeed. Organizations such as Weight Watchers seem to have enormous success, and joining the ranks can certainly do no harm and will frequently do a great deal of good.

## The cholesterol problem

Overweight is frequently associated with other potent risk factors, particularly diabetes and high blood pressure. If these two are eliminated (which can be done), it may be that the increased tendency to atherosclerosis is due to a high animal fat content in the diet rather than to simple overweight. With widespread affluence there has been an increase in the consumption of all animal products. The fat in animal food products is not only butter, cheese and the fat on steak or a rasher of bacon, but the invisible fats in all animal products – even eggs, milk and lean beef have at least 10 per cent fat.

Having said that, the story then becomes a bit more complicated. About 90 per cent of fat is made up of fatty acids; some of these are 'essential' to the body, others are 'non-essential' and are used as energy stores. Fatty acids are divided into saturated and non-saturated – the more hydrogen atoms present, the more saturated, thus 2 or more hydrogen atoms = polysaturated, 1 or fewer hydrogen atoms = monosaturated. Saturated fats are generally solid at room temperature, for example lard and butter; unsaturated fats are liquid at room temperature, corn and sunflower oil, for instance; this is because the former come from warm-blooded animals – the fats are then liquid at body temperatures – the others from fish and plants which have lower temperatures.

Cholesterol is a special form of fat which does not contain a fatty acid; it is made in the liver and travels in the blood to parts of the body where it is needed, such as the brain and sex hormones. A small amount of dietary cholesterol is needed – about 1 per cent of the total weight of fat in the diet. The body makes about 30 grams of cholesterol a month but the average diet contains about 7 grams excess per month. It is thought that the saturated fat and extra cholesterol in animal fats in some way impairs the body's regulation of cholesterol and that the surplus enters the bloodstream; a fatty streak develops on the wall of an artery which ulcerates, scars and forms an atheroscleritic plaque. Up to the scarring, this process is reversible, but if the plaque enlarges and turbulence in the blood flow causes a clot to form on the plaque, the bore of the vessel is reduced even more and the reduced blood flow starves the muscle of oxygen. In the heart muscle this starvation may manifest itself as angina; if a piece of clot breaks off, the vessel may become completely blocked and result in a heart attack.

In the Western world, countries consuming little dietary cholesterol have a low incidence of heart disease, those with a high consumption have high levels. It would seem that the main factor in plaque formation is the level of cholesterol in the bloodstream, therefore the less cholesterol and the more unsaturated fats in the diet, the better.

Cholesterol is one of the fatty materials in the blood called lipids; there are other lipids known as triglycerides. Across the world it would appear that where blood lipids in general are low, there is a low incidence of atherosclerosis and heart disease. If the level of cholesterol in the blood is high the risk of heart trouble increases more than if the triglycerides are high.

It has recently been discovered that cholesterol is transported in the body by a chemical called lipoprotein. Low density lipoprotein (LDL) carries cholesterol from the liver to the body cells where it is used in the making of cell membranes, hormones, etc., while lipoproteins of a higher density (HDL) transport unused cholesterol back to the liver for excretion from the body. It appears that if high blood cholesterol is linked to high levels of LDL there is a greater risk of developing ischaemic heart disease; on the other hand where high cholesterol levels are linked to high density lipoproteins, the risk is decreased. Thus there seems to be some sort of protective element in high levels of HDL.

Tests can be made on the blood to find the levels of HDL and LDL, and the ratio of one to the other can be estimated. These levels are affected favourably by exercise, weight reducing and low cholesterol diets, and unfavourably by smoking and inactivity.

The cholesterol and triglyceride levels in the blood vary and are classified as being within normal limits or as abnormal. Dr. D. S. Fredrickson, an American, has classified them as follows:

Type 1. *Cholesterol slightly elevated – triglycerides grossly elevated.* Fairly rare.

Type 2. *Cholesterol elevated – triglycerides normal.* More common.

Type 3. *Cholesterol and triglycerides both elevated.* Fairly rare.

Type 4. *Cholesterol normal – triglycerides elevated.* Most common.

Type 5. *Cholesterol normal – triglycerides grossly elevated.* Fairly rare.

Elevated triglyceride levels can be a hereditary tendency, but more frequently they are associated with obesity and should fall if a weight-reducing diet is followed – sugar and alcohol have been specifically incriminated so the intake of these should be particularly curbed.

## Personality type

A great deal of work is being done to try and find out if there is a 'heart attack' personality. For some years these have been classified as Type A and Type B; Type A is the so-called time-addict, a competitive, ambitious, aggressive, impatient type who is usually working to a tight schedule, is always in a rush, often over-committed, has a habit of interjecting and carrying on finger-wagging conversations. Type B is the more casual, phlegmatic kind of individual, much more easygoing. Not surprisingly the Type A person appears to have a much higher chance of a heart attack. After this first simple classification, however, sub-divisions are now appearing as work continues to help predict the occurrence of heart disease.

## Diabetes

Diabetes is associated with increased levels of sugar in the blood and is often accompanied by an imbalance of blood fats. The problems that this can produce in the circulation may show at an early age. In people under 45 years, the incidence of heart disease for both men and women with diabetes is six times higher than for those without. Why this is so is not yet very clear; such patients commonly have high blood fat levels, but this cannot be the complete answer as diabetics in Japan, the Middle East and North Africa don't seem to carry the same risk as those in the Western world.

## Inadequate exercise

To an unfit, overweight, middle-aged television addict the very thought of taking exercise is almost enough to produce a heart attack. Exercise to the unfit is a grim and unattractive pastime. Again, the medical profession is divided as to the importance of exercise. The largest study of any community to date – in Framingham, USA, which has been carefully monitored for many years with particular reference to heart disease – suggests that the 'risk of death in least physically active males is three times higher than more active males', and experiments with animals show that mild to moderate exercise does increase the size of the blood vessel system in the heart. Some would disagree with these statements, but most agree that exercise is beneficial.

The body is a great supply and demand machine; it only does as much as it has to do. If muscles aren't used they get smaller and weaker. This can be seen quite dramatically in the muscles of the thigh after a cartilage operation; wasting can be seen within days of the operation if muscle-building exercises are not started to prevent it. So people who exercise generally feel well, eat well and look well. The muscles are strong and efficient; the heart which is asked to beat faster and stronger in exercise conditions has good tone and reserve, with an efficient blood supply; the circulation works well, and the small vessels, which remain closed when not required, work smoothly if called upon; joints which are put through their full range of movements, work well. If a door is left shut for years it will be creaky when you open it – leave a joint dormant and the same thing will happen.

Nobody of course is suggesting that the TV addict should run a marathon every day of the week. Even a small amount of exercise is enough as long as it is done regularly; it could be following one of the standard books of physical fitness programmes, jogging, cycling or going up and down on a step, according to personal preference. Thirty to forty minutes divided into three sessions over a week is considered sufficient, and once the first stage has been overcome and general fitness improves, exercise becomes a pleasure and sports like tennis and swimming can be enjoyed even into old age.

Exercise has to be sufficiently demanding to cause puffing – a round of golf, for example, although relaxing, can hardly be defined as exercise. There are two types of exercise: isometric, which builds the muscles, and isotonic (dynamic), which includes sport and athletics. It is the latter which is good for the heart.

## Stress

How any one person reacts to a given set of circumstances is as variable as people themselves. Stimulation is a healthy and pleasurable emotion. The body can, like a machine, be put under stress and pressure and providing this is within acceptable limits, like a machine it will respond and run smoothly and efficiently. The stress may be physical as in exercise, or psychological or emotional – the body's response to either is identical.

The way the body reacts to these stresses can be measured by the heart rate and blood pressure response.

In periods of physical and emotional pressure these responses increase and prepare the body for action – whatever that may be. Part of this response is chemical: sugar, fat, cholesterol and clotting elements in the blood will all increase, and the body becomes a highly charged machine ready for 'fight or flight'.

Trouble really starts when the body is in this highly charged state all the time. Tables have been produced giving points for various pressures; bankruptcy, divorce, family death, a sudden change in circumstances are but a few of the classic examples causing constant pressure and resulting in a constantly raised heart rate, blood pressure and blood cholesterol, which are major factors in plaque development and atherosclerosis. Often these are the circumstances in which people will seek relief in cigarettes, thus raising heart rate and blood pressure still further.

It is worth knowing some of the warning signs for this highly charged state developing. The limits are governed by the personality, a stressful lifestyle – often self-generated – and the ability of the body to cope with both of these, and will show themselves in various ways: changes in appetite (up or down), changes in sleep pattern (difficulty in going to sleep or early waking), general malaise and weakness, loss of sex drive and associated problems, inability to relax, irritability, not being able to cope, feelings of family and work mates not cooperating, loss of sense of humour, feelings of despair and failure, inability to concentrate, loss of efficiency, inability to complete one job at a time, fear of disease and death – these are only a few of the pointers out of the enormous lists that have been made. Of course most people will recognize themselves in a few of these categories, but if reasonable insight into personality and lifestyle adds up to a fair score of them, then steps should be taken to reduce the risk.

## Levels of stress

| Events | Scale of impact | | |
|---|---|---|---|
| Death of spouse | 100 | Son or daughter leaving home | 29 |
| Divorce | 73 | Trouble with in-laws | 29 |
| Marital separation | 65 | Major personal achievement | 28 |
| Jail term | 63 | Change in spouse's work | 26 |
| Death of close family member | 63 | Starting or leaving school | 26 |
| Personal injury or illness | 53 | Change in living conditions | 25 |
| Marriage | 50 | Revision of personal habits | 24 |
| Loss of job | 47 | Trouble with boss | 23 |
| Marital reconciliation | 45 | Change in work hours | 20 |
| Retirement | 45 | Change in residence | 20 |
| Health problems in family | 44 | Change in schools | 20 |
| Pregnancy | 40 | Change in recreation | 19 |
| Sex difficulties | 39 | Change in church activities | 19 |
| Gain of new family member | 39 | Change in social activities | 18 |
| Business readjustment | 39 | Small mortgage taken out | 17 |
| Change in financial state | 38 | Change in sleeping habits | 16 |
| Death of a close friend | 37 | Change in family reunions | 15 |
| Change in line of work | 36 | Change in eating habits | 15 |
| More arguments with spouse | 35 | Vacation | 13 |
| Large mortgage taken out | 31 | Christmas | 12 |
| Foreclosure of mortgage | 30 | Minor violations of the law | 11 |
| Change in work status | 29 | | |

*If you score more than 150 points during the last six months you are under stress, and your chances of becoming ill are much greater than normal.*

As I said at the beginning of this chapter, these are not the only risk factors but they are the ones most generally accepted. If I included all those postulated by research papers and institutes, you would wonder how anybody could possibly survive their three score years and ten. There is no doubt, however, that the presence of any of the factors mentioned here increases the risk of heart attack, a risk that a gambler may be prepared to take, but the more factors present the shorter the odds. If you have three factors present – smoking, high blood cholesterol and un-

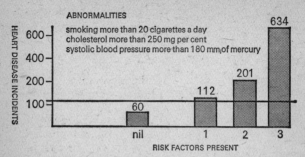

*A diagram showing the effect of multiple risk factors. The chances of developing coronary artery disease rise steeply with the addition of each factor.*

treated high blood pressure, for example, then your chances are six times higher than if you had only one, and ten times higher than if you had none.

Yet with the minimum of self-care, a little imagination, and a great deal of cooperation and will power, most of these risks can be eliminated. High blood pressure can be controlled with regular medication as more and more preparations become available. The same applies to a raised level of blood cholesterol. Keeping the intake of animal fats at a low level will often eliminate this potent factor, and very high levels of cholesterol, perhaps a disorder of cholesterol metabolism (which sometimes runs in families), can be treated by regular medication.

It is difficult to change your personality – and not always desirable – but almost all of us, if we really want to, can alter our schedules and commitments to relieve chronic stress and the damage it causes. The prospect of taking real regular exercise may not seem too attractive, but once you have made the initial move it's not really so bad, and you may even find it enjoyable. Certainly physically fit people feel well, besides the added bonus of eliminating another risk factor.

For many of us, the two factors most difficult to eradicate are the enjoyable pastimes of eating and smoking, and, as I have said, too often the motivation to control these is the shock of a heart attack. It seems a pity that the writing has to be in such large letters before it is read. Nicotine is a powerful stimulant, but giving it up should not be an unsurmountable problem with the maximum of will power. The food addict has a similar problem, from which there is no easy way out; there are several tablets which are supposed to lower the appetite but they are not generally successful, and again the only way is the hard one – make the decision to lose weight and stick to it.

If proof is still needed that these factors are not a lot of rubbish, the following story may be convincing. During the war in Korea autopsies were carried out on some of the all-American boys who had been well fed with animal fats, had driven around in cars from the age of 16, and smoked like the troopers they were. It was found that a notably high percentage of these apparently fit young men showed extensive evidence of atherosclerosis in the heart vessels. A nation-wide education programme in primary prevention was begun: jogging became a cult, cholesterol was closely watched, heart health education was widespread. And the result? The incidence of coronary artery disease in America is falling – not just a little, but by a very significant amount. The unfortunate young American soldiers who were killed in the Vietnam war and on whom autopsy was performed, showed very little evidence of atherosclerosis in the heart vessels.

Is the same thing happening in Britain? Not in the field of primary prevention anyway; there is considerable apathy about the whole problem and the incidence of coronary artery disease is still increasing at an alarming rate.

# 3 Chest Pain: Angina and Heart Attacks

Just what happens in a heart attack? And in the pain known as angina? Both are the result of a blockage (or in the case of angina, partial blockage) in the coronary arteries (the blood vessels supplying the heart) and their branches, caused by *atheroma* (see page 17) and resulting in an inadequate supply of oxygen and essential nutrients to the heart muscle; the area supplied by the affected vessels will become inefficient and eventually the strong and mobile muscle, deprived of adequate nourishment, will become rigid and inelastic.

The result of this process will usually be pain (see page 38), varying in character according to the position and extent of damaged tissue; often the type of pain will indicate what sort of damage has occurred. When angina is occurring, the use of ever more ingenious methods of investigation – such as exercise electrocardiography and blood analysis – now makes it possible to define, with increasing accuracy, just what is going on. The damage may be so slight, however, that it could only be detected by a microscope.

The progressive disease process caused by atheroma is increasing in incidence, especially in the Western world.

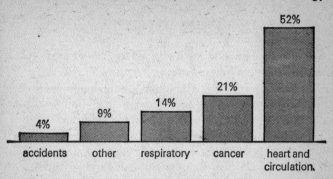

*Causes of death in Great Britain. Over half the total is accounted for by diseases of the heart and circulation, less than a quarter by cancer.*

The approximate number of people who die annually from this disease in Great Britain at this time is 150,000, yet in the early 1940s the figure was nearer 18,500. By the 1960s it had risen to 100,000 and the current figure represents more than twice the number of people dying each year from all forms of cancer. Of course, there are factors that make these figures look over-pessimistic – an increasing population with an increasing life-expectancy and consequent rise in the age of the population, and more accurate diagnostic equipment available to doctors – but the trend is there, not only in Great Britain but in all countries that keep medical statistics. It should not be underestimated. To have really accurate figures for the incidence of this disease, 'heart events' would have to be made notifiable – like measles – as many, many people survive a heart attack and die from some other cause. There are those who believe that this figure would reach something like 1,000,000 cases per year; even if that proves to be something of an exaggeration, it remains a colossal problem and anything that can be done to reduce it is worth spending money on.

# Angina pectoris

The term angina pectoris is derived from two Latin words: *angere*, to strangle or suffocate, and *pectus*, the chest. It was first used by William Haberden, the eighteenth-century English physician, in 1768, to describe the strangling sensation which is frequently present in this condition.

Angina is caused by a deficiency in the oxygen supply to the heart muscle, usually due to atheroma of the arteries reducing the bore of the vessel. It can also be the result of other diseases such as anaemia, where the vessel may be normal but the oxygen supply reduced through a decrease in the number of red blood cells which carry the oxygen. Typically, the pain occurs when the oxygen demand is raised above basic requirements, such as at exercise; if angina occurs at rest it is due to – and known as – acute coronary insufficiency.

The factors that most often bring on an attack of angina are as follows.

1. Physical effort which demands increased output from the heart: walking uphill or even a gradual slope, which may start the pain more easily than walking upstairs.

2. Extremes of temperature, particularly cold – hurrying against a cold wind, entering a cold bedroom, even getting between cold sheets. Cold air causes the vessels in the lungs to constrict, reducing the amount of oxygen uptake.

3. Large meals cause supplies of blood to be shunted to the intestines, where it is needed for the digestive process.

4. Emotion – frustration, marital rows or excitement, watching sport, unpleasant dreams – demands an increase in cardiac output as a result of adrenalin secretion.

## What sort of pain – and where?

Classically the pain of angina is behind the breast bone,

running the length of the bone and spreading across the chest; it may be referred up to the throat (hence the name) and up to the jaw and teeth – often throwing suspicion on an illfitting denture if it happens after a heavy meal. Sometimes the pain is referred to the armpits and down the arm – more frequently on the left side – to the elbow and even to the fingers; at other times the only pain at the onset is in these areas away from the breast bone – perhaps only in the jaw or elbow – but sooner or later the breast bone becomes involved. On other occasions there may be no pain at all, but a feeling of heaviness in the arms or chest, with tingling in the fingers. It has been known for pain to be referred to a diseased site – a bad tooth or an arthritic shoulder – and quite often attention is focused on an effect rather than the cause. At times the pain may be so insignificant that there is no intimation of the real cause.

There are many classical expressions used to describe angina – patients attempting to relate the character of the pain or sensation will often use the same expression, and this can provide clues to the origin of the problem.

One of the world's leading heart specialists, Dr Samuel Oram, in his book *Clinical Heart Disease*, gives a list of these typical descriptions, which includes:

| | |
|---|---|
| Pressure | Made me sweat |
| Heaviness | Severe heartburn |
| Tightness | Squeezing |
| Constricting | Tight band |
| Indigestion | Soreness |
| Bursting | Vice-like |
| Like a lump that's stuck | Fear of impending death |
| Discomfort – not a pain | Bursting outwards |
| Unpleasant – difficult to describe | Like a ball being pushed through a tube too small for it |
| Excruciating | |

These Dr Oram considers to be pains or sensations suggestive of angina; the following list is of descriptions which will almost certainly *exclude* a heart origin:

| | |
|---|---|
| Stabbing | Piercing |
| Pricking | Like a stitch |
| Niggling | Sharp jab |
| Shooting | Cutting |
| Burning | Stinging |
| Knifelike | |

Angina is not a dramatic event, but the pain will usually pull the victim up short, for the oxygen debt to the heart must be repaid. So slackening the pace, whether of movement or emotion – resting for a few minutes – eases the pain, which will usually pass quite quickly. To compare the heart with an engine once more, if an engine with a faulty fuel supply is allowed to work within reasonable limits it will do so quite efficiently – but put an added load on to it (e.g. put your foot down on the accelerator) and the fuel will not arrive fast enough so the engine starts to misfire; if you take your foot off the accelerator the engine will fire evenly again. This is exactly what happens to the heart in angina – when you exert yourself the poor fuel supply results in fuel starvation which causes pain in the characteristic ways already described; reduce the activity and the pain will go.

## Treatment for angina

In the case of a motor car, it would not be difficult to disconnect the fuel supply, blow the pipes out, clean out the carburettor and put it all together again with the problem solved. Not so easy to do this with a human heart, but there are several courses open which although not curing the condition will certainly help to relieve the pain. The first and most obvious way to avoid angina would be to adopt a lifestyle utterly devoid of any activity likely to start the pain. This would mean *total* inactivity, no emotional stress, no physical stress, an even temperature and no stimulation of any kind – in other words an existence rather than a life, not acceptable to most people and quite unnecessary. Perhaps the most demoralizing part of this whole disease is fear of the unknown and a lack of information about what the future will be. With good, controlled, informed advice a high quality of life should be possible.

Living with angina demands that one should cut one's coat according to the cloth. Most people will be able to continue in their employment, although obviously some jobs will be unsuitable. Long hours involving hard physical work may become impossible, and not only physical jobs present problems – people such as airline pilots and train drivers will have to find alternative work, as much for the sake of those for whom they are responsible as for themselves. In general, however, to give up an occupation of many years and start again at something new, may present even greater problems in the way of financial insecurity and lack of confidence.

Vigorous, competitive sport will generally produce angina so may not be advisable, but physical activity that is less demanding should be encouraged – walking, golf, swimming and so on, as much as can be done without producing excessive symptoms. Life may be lived to the limit but not beyond it. It is frequently the case that when physical activity is increased – such as in a programme of controlled exercise (see Chapter 7) – the onset of angina is delayed, and consequently the range of activity possible increases and morale and confidence improve.

Exercise is not the only answer, of course. A great deal of angina is the result of bad habits acquired early and sustained over many years, so these have to be dealt with – it

is pointless to deal with the angina then sit back and let
the precipitating causes relentlessly continue. The havoc
that tobacco smoking causes to the heart has been discussed at length in Chapter 2, but for those who still have
any doubts the diagram below should be overwhelming.
Without going into too much detail here on the reading of
an electrocardiogram, it can be clearly seen that the wave

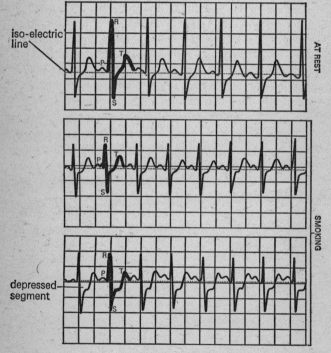

*Nicotine has a very powerful effect on the heart and its circulation. The
top trace is normal, but on the lower traces it can be seen how smoking
progressively increases the rate and the line shape changes (sags) showing
that the heart muscle is starved of oxygen.*

pattern changes with smoking. The characteristic 'sag' is the electrical manifestation of the heart muscle being starved of oxygen, and is directly comparable to the change in shape seen at exercise with angina (see page 82).

There are other causes of angina to be avoided. One is well described by the Americanism 'hassle', and covers a multitude of sins: arguments, disagreements, frustrations, emotional stresses. These are probably as difficult to avoid as a packet of cigarettes, but it is well worth making a positive, conscious effort to avoid such situations.

The effects of a diet high in animal fats and cholesterol have already been discussed, so it will be obvious that if the pump – the power behind the circulation – is showing signs of fuel starvation – angina – by having to drive blood around a body considerably heavier than it was designed to be, this effort will produce a further strain on an already overworked heart. The commonest cause of overweight is too much food. If you eat more than your body requires over a period of several years, the excess will be converted and stored as fat. The only way to lose this is to reduce the food intake to such a level that the fat is broken down and used up. Losing weight, like giving up smoking, requires a tremendous amount of self-discipline but it is well worth the effort.

If you are faced with the unpleasant prospect of giving up these long-indulged habits, it is sensible not to try and do so all at the same time. Most people who give up smoking will compensate by putting something else in their mouths for a while, frequently sweets, and will therefore put on more weight. It is much more important to stop smoking, and once that is conquered you can start the weight losing. The physical activity – regular exercise – can continue through both the other battles and indeed may well be a help in them.

# Drugs

So far I have talked about angina and the responsibility of the patient, but the physician does have a large range of drugs available which will relieve the symptom of angina. Some of these may be taken regularly on a calculated basis, others are carried around by the patient and taken when the pain occurs; these will relieve the pain very quickly and may be taken prior to any activity that is known to bring on angina.

Without going into a detailed list of these drugs and comparing their beneficial properties, they can be divided into two main groups. The fast-acting ones cause a dilatation of the vessels of the heart and a reduction in resistance to the flow of blood in the circulation; this reduces the work of the heart by reducing the load on the pump and allows the circulating fuel to be used more efficiently, thus relieving the fuel starvation and the pain. These tablets are either designed to be placed under the tongue, which allows a rapid absorption as they are sucked, or made with a slowly dispersing action which will last for several hours.

The second group, known as beta-blocking drugs, is now very large (they are discussed more fully on page 71). These work on the sympathetic nerve supply to the heart, and by 'blocking' their action they reduce the heart rate, which reduces the output and brings down the blood pressure. The oxygen requirement to the heart muscle is approximately proportional to the heart rate, so preventing a rapid heart rate which may develop in exercise or emotion is of great benefit. Taking one of these drugs regularly will improve exercise tolerance – that is, the ability to perform physical work – and reduce angina.

Like all useful and effective drugs they are not without some side-effects, but there is now such a wide choice available that in cases where such effects do occur, an alternative can usually be found. Drugs will be dealt with in more detail in Chapter 4.

## Surgery

Great advances are being made all the time in the field of surgery (discussed at length in Chapter 6), though it is still a subject of discussion and controversy. In Great Britain, as a general rule, 'by-pass' surgery (see page 98) is only undertaken after extensive investigation, and in some cases the rigorous criteria for surgery will not be filled even if medical treatment has not been successful – that is, in spite of increasing dosage of tablets, quality of life continues to deteriorate, with decreasing activity and increasing angina. With careful selection and good surgery, however, this operation is now safe and effective, with an almost miraculous transformation of lifestyle in most cases.

# Heart attacks

I have described the partial obstruction to the flow of blood along the vessel which occurs in angina; in a heart attack the obstruction is complete, and the area of heart muscle supplied by the blocked vessel is completely starved of fuel and will die.

Exactly what happens and how in coronary artery thrombosis is still – surprisingly, in view of how common it is – a subject of considerable argument and speculation. The picture is slowly beginning to clarify, however. For many years it was thought that there was a single cause: that a clot of blood (*thrombus*) formed in one of the vessels of the heart, detached itself from the wall and moved along the vessel, eventually reaching the smaller vessels; these were too small to allow it to move any further, so there it stuck, blocking any further blood flow to that part of the heart muscle supplied by the particular vessel and starving it of fuel. Result – a 'heart attack'.

Further research suggested that the clot was not in fact the primary cause but was part of some other process which itself caused an acute, fast obstruction. This work was much discussed and argued over, and has now developed into another theory which may well turn out to be the answer. This involves the formation of atheromatous plaques (see page 17), which are often found stuck to the wall of ageing heart vessels. The plaque cracks and a split appears into which the blood flows, causing a bleed in the wall of the coronary artery. This produces the normal reaction of blood to haemorrhage: tiny cells called *platelets*, when in contact with damaged cells, become sticky and band together to try and stop any further blood loss. When this happens in the artery wall, the bunch of platelets – a *platelet thrombus* – extends from the crack in the plaque out into the blood vessel and blocks the blood flow. Thus the clot is the secondary result of the primary cause, which is the opening of the crack in the atheromotous plaque already on the vessel wall.

This all sounds quite logical, but if we go into it a little more we will find complications. Why do the platelets stick together? Because they come into contact with tough, fibrous tissue in the vessel wall called *collagen*, and this triggers off the massing of the platelets. But if an artificial blood vessel – now made of Teflon, of non-stick saucepan fame – which has no collagen, is punctured, an exactly similar process of platelet massing and plugging results; so some other mechanism than the collagen must be working. The latest theory is that the red blood cells have unusually severe forces to deal with at the site of small haemorrhages or punctures in the vessel wall (especially in vessels which have atheromatous plaques), and to cope with these increased forces the red cells produce agents which increase the massing of the platelets. It has been shown in a research programme that platelets flowing past a defect at tremendous speed manage to plug the damage at a rate of 10,000 platelets a second – almost 1 million a minute! If this process of massing platelets could be slowed down, the small bleed into the vessel wall could become relatively harmless, that is without the extension into the vessel itself and the resulting splitting off of the thrombus to cause a complete obstruction.

There is at present a great deal of interest in and development of drugs that are capable of inhibiting the massing of platelets, and results of trials so far are encouraging. It may be that with the long-term use of these drugs, the incidence of recurrent heart attacks will be greatly reduced.

## What happens in a heart attack?

The magnitude of the catastrophe of a heart attack depends very much on which vessel is involved and the age and general health of the individual involved. Using the analogy of road systems again, it is obviously less harmful if a small B-type road is blocked than one of the main motorways, since a blockage on one of them would in turn starve the A roads and B roads which would involve a considerable area of the heart muscle.

The centres controlling the electrical system of the heart, the *sino-atrial node* and the *atrio-ventricular node*, most frequently gain their blood supply from the right coronary artery (the anatomy of the coronary artery circulation is described in Chapter 1), and if one of these small branches to the system becomes blocked, rhythm disturbances may result and rapid treatment may be necessary to correct them.

The body is a very good self-healing mechanism, and although the scar on the vessel wall will always remain – as scars on the skin do – attempts are made by the circulation to create an alternative route and open up small vessels to form a collateral circulation.

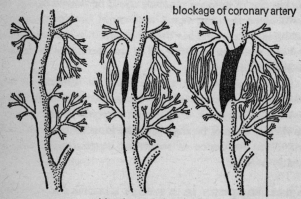

blockage of coronary artery

blood vessels forming a collateral circulation

*Collateral circulation. There is present in normal tissue an intricate network of blood vessels; if a major vessel becomes obstructed, this network attempts to assist the reduced passage of blood by forming an alternative route. As is shown in the diagram, the collateral supply increases to keep pace with the blockage. These changes can be seen on angiograms.*

## What can bring on a heart attack?

Causes are similar to those which can bring on an attack of angina – unaccustomed exercise, anger, frustration, cold, heavy meals; but unlike angina, heart attacks commonly occur at rest, often waking the person up. Other less common causes are shock, haemorrhage, anaesthetics or even a surgical operation.

## What does it feel like?

About one third of people who have a heart attack will be suffering from angina or have experienced it in the past, and it may have increased in frequency and severity before the attack. But in about 65 per cent of 'heart attacks' the individual has never had any problem relating to the chest.

The pain is frequently sudden in onset, and feels much the same as that described for angina. It may vary from being very severe – 'like an oak tree lying across my chest' – to merely an ache in the arm. Unlike angina, the pain persists and will not be relieved by pills that were effective in angina. As a general rule of thumb, any pain in the area of the chest such as is described in the list on page 39 which persists for longer than 30 minutes should be regarded as a heart attack until proved otherwise. Frequently the pain is accompanied by a feeling of impending death which has not been experienced before.

The pain is usually in the middle of the breast bone but can be higher or lower; often it radiates to one or both sides of the chest, sometimes up into the neck or lower jaw and to one or both arms – this is often described as a feeling of heaviness in the arms and may be accompanied by numbness or tingling in the hands and fingers. With the pain there may be other complaints such as sweating, faintness, giddiness, difficulty in breathing, a feeling of sickness, sometimes even vomiting. These are common sensations at the onset of a heart attack, but routine investigations of healthy people have provided clear evidence that an individual has suffered a heart attack and been completely unaware of it – probably dismissed it as an attack of indigestion or feeling under par. There are no figures of how often this happens, but it is certainly not a rare finding.

Patients in pain are often in distress, pale, cold and

sweating. There may be changes in the rate of the heart-beat: faster, called *tachycardia*, and slower, *bradycardia*. The blood pressure may rise, *hypertension*, or fall, *hypotension*. There may be transient shock – changes which are a result of the body's reaction to pain – and in this case a rapid improvement is seen after administration of a pain-killing drug, so that within a few hours the patient may look and feel normal.

Sudden death from a heart attack usually occurs within the first two hours after the onset of symptoms (it is claimed that out of a quarter of a million people suffering heart attacks almost half of those who died did so within the first two hours) so it is very important to seek medical aid without delay if you suspect a heart attack has occurred. Delay over a matter of hours could make all the difference to survival, and a doctor would much rather see a patient with chest pain that turns out to be indigestion than have to attend somebody who has delayed calling for help for too long. The question of whether it is preferable to be treated at home or in hospital will depend on a number of factors which are discussed more fully in the next chapter.

# 4 What Happens in a Heart Attack

What should you do if you suspect you are having a heart attack? Or if your loved one or colleague is having a heart attack? Whom should you call? And when? The answer in every case is – don't sit and wait, call the doctor or an ambulance immediately.

In Great Britain we are fortunate to have a general practitioner service, with doctors prepared to visit us at home. This is by no means a worldwide privilege. In the United States and Canada, for instance, the attitude is that if a heart attack is suspected the patient should be taken to the expert and his equipment in hospital rather than be visited at home. Both systems have their advantages and disadvantages.

But let us assume that the doctor is prepared to visit at home. First he will make his examination. He has to make a major decision: should the patient be admitted to hospital or kept at home? In doing so he will take into consideration the general condition of the patient; he will decide whether he is 'shocked' or not from the rhythm and character of the pulse and the blood pressure – this may fall considerably in a heart attack and constant checking may be necessary. He will also take into account the patient's history, if this is known to him. He will examine the neck. There may be visible changes which tell him the heart is beginning to 'fail', in which case the veins in the neck become prominent. He will then examine the heart with his stethoscope. This will tell him the rhythm. Sometimes he may hear a sound like a galloping horse, or a noise called a 'rub', which tells him that the coverings of the heart are irritated. Next he will examine the lungs. It may be that some fluid is accumulating at the bottom of them, and this will be associated with some shortness of breath which is made worse by any movement. Lastly he will examine the ankles. These may be normal, but they could be swollen, suggesting that there has been trouble for some time.

If the doctor decides that the patient is in good condition and has no apparent complications, he may decide to keep him at home. This would be most likely if the patient is over 60 years old. (There has been some evidence lately that the older age group particularly respond better when treated at home rather than in hospital.) In this case the doctor has a considerable commitment to visit and treat. The home environment, family circumstances and family cooperation are of course of paramount importance, and no one would consider keeping a patient at home if he were living by himself with a lavatory at the bottom of the garden.

Relief of pain is the most important facet of treatment at this stage, and if the doctor decides to keep the patient at home arrangements have to be made for either himself or the district nurse to visit at least two or three times a day for the first few days, to keep any pain at bay with pain-killing injections. The patient should be kept in bed until the pain has gone, using a bottle or bedpan. Then, providing the lavatory is easily accessible, he may get up to use it within twenty-four hours of being pain free – no stairs though.

As far as my own rule of thumb is concerned, anyone of 60 years or over is treated at home if at all possible, and anyone of 45 years or less is admitted to hospital. The 45–60 year olds are treated individually on their own merits, but if in any doubt I normally refer them for admission to the local hospital.

All this assumes that the heart attack happens at home. In fact most heart attacks do seem to occur there. A trial from Nottingham found that 75 per cent happened at home, and in about two-thirds of these the family doctor was called rather than an ambulance. If the heart attack does happen outside the protective environment of the home, it is more than likely that the choice of home treatment or hospitalization will not occur – the ambulance will be summoned.

What then should you do if you come into contact with somebody you suspect is having a heart attack? It cannot be reiterated often enough that the dangers are most extreme in the first two hours. If in any doubt, call an ambulance.

For some time in the United States and more recently in a few isolated centres in this country, there have been highly trained crews manning ambulances to deal with emergencies which may include heart attacks. Just how effective such ambulances are is open to question, and they are extremely expensive to run – not only in terms of equipment but of adequately trained staff to run them. In any event, they are not yet a standard part of British medicine.

Assuming that a heart attack is suspected, whether confirmed by a doctor who decides that admission to hospital is necessary or whether an ambulance is called by a member of the general public, what happens next? How will the patient cope with the white-coated jungle which is likely to be so new to him?

In ideal circumstances the ambulance will arrive at the admitting section of the hospital or the casualty department. If the staff have been given advance warning of a suspected heart attack, the wheels of admission should run like clockwork: out of the ambulance on to a trolley, into a lift if necessary, and then straight into bed.

Unfortunately this is not always the case. When the well-known comedian Eric Morecambe suffered a heart attack, he was driving his car at the time. It was late at night and he did not know what was happening, so he stopped and asked a man in the street to drive him to the nearest hospital. Once there it was some time before he got past the reception desk and was laid on a trolley. He was then asked to give his name, age, address, etc. and finally, before being taken to bed, he had to give his autograph to the man who had driven him there! This event did have a happy ending, but it was during those crucial minutes that very severe complications could have occurred.

So, assuming the barrier of admission has been crossed and you are safely in bed, what sort of place are you likely to find yourself in?

Over the past fifteen years special wards called intensive care units have become part of most large hospitals. Their name describes exactly what they are: small wards designed to give patients intensive care and nursing. Such units have a huge array of equipment and are manned by highly trained nursing staff – the ratio is frequently one nurse per bed in these wards. They are specifically for patients (not only those suffering from heart attacks) who require constant observation and whose condition may change rapidly. Some hospitals have what is called a coronary care unit, which specializes in monitoring and treating patients suffering from heart problems of one sort or another, but mainly heart attacks.

If an intensive (or coronary) care unit is available in the hospital to which you are taken, that is where you will find yourself. What will happen next?

The doctor in charge of such a unit is usually a senior house officer who lives in the hospital or very close to it, so that he is readily available should he be required in an emergency. He is not working single-handed and can call upon further specialist help if necessary, but it is likely that a doctor of this grade will visit you soon after admission.

The patient with a suspected heart attack arriving at the unit may have anything from a mild pain to acute pain and shock requiring much skilled medical expertise in the minimum of time to give him the best chance of survival. For the purposes of this chapter let us take two heart attack patients, one whose recovery should be automatic and uneventful, and one who will require treatment with the battery of equipment available.

# The uncomplicated heart attack

Immediately after being settled into bed in the coronary care unit, the patient will be linked to a 'monitor'. This is a screen which looks like a small television set, usually above the bed. The link is obtained by sticking small electrodes to the chest with adhesive collars, a totally painless procedure. The monitor shows the electrical activity of the heart by scanning across the screen. It is important to keep a very close watch on the heart, particularly during the first twenty-four hours after admission as it is during this time that the damaged heart can produce the rhythm disturbances which may require urgent attention. These monitors around the ward are linked to a central console, like an island in the middle of the room, where a screen displays what is going on at each bed. Thus the nursing staff can observe each patient's heart activity without prowling around all the time.

## Filling in the background

The doctor in charge of the unit will then visit, and it is he who will decide on the immediate treatment. If the patient is comfortable and in a good condition, he will take down his medical history and make a full examination. He will want an account of the events leading up to the time of calling for help. He will question in detail the type of pain experienced, where it was, whether it was of gradual or sudden onset. Did it stay where it was or move? Did it radiate anywhere, particularly the shoulders or arms, neck or throat? Did it cause shortness of breath? Had a pain like this ever happened before? He will ask whether any discomfort has been experienced in the past with exertion or after heavy meals, and whether there is any history of fainting or waking at night breathless.

As the patient describes the pain, the doctor will try to discover how severe it was. This is of course a very variable sensation as some people can tolerate pain better than others, but there are certain characteristics of pain which suggest the heart as their origin. The doctor will ask about the duration of the pain and what affected it: was it worse or better with movement, did breathing make it worse, and so on. All these questions, although unable to provide a diagnosis in themselves, will, together with the findings of the examination, build up a picture which should lead to accurate diagnosis.

Enquiries are also made into the patient's past medical record: whether there have been previous admissions to hospital or prolonged treatment of any sort.

Having gone into the history of the present complaint in detail, the patient's general health then comes under scrutiny. Has the appetite been good or bad? If bad, in what way? Has there been intolerance of any particular food such as fats, which may suggest a different illness such as gall bladder disease. Is the weight steady? Most people do not weigh themselves regularly, and a useful guide is whether there has been any change in the fit of a person's clothes – are they appearing to get larger or smaller? The bowel habits and passing of urine are enquired after, and the menstrual cycle in women.

Sleep patterns are important. If there has been a change in sleeping habits – either difficulty in getting off to sleep or early waking – when previously the patient has slept well, this can be suggestive of an anxiety or depression state which may have some bearing on the situation. If there has been a change, the reason should be sought. Has the patient been under pressure in business, family or financial affairs? If so for how long, and are the problems likely to be resolved? Is he under constant stress and pressure at work? Do threats of redundancy exist, or does he feel under- or over-promoted?

Does the patient smoke? If he does, in what form? If it is cigarettes, how many a day and for how many years? Most people who smoke cigarettes tend to be slightly ashamed of the fact, and as a rule underestimate the number. Having been given a negative answer the doctor, on digging a little further, often discovers that the patient smoked 40 cigarettes a day and decided to give up just the week before – hardly long enough for the system to have gained any benefit at all.

The doctor will want to know how much the patient is in the habit of drinking, and what tablets he is taking (or has taken recently). The latter is very important, as it may affect any treatment that is decided upon. If anti-depressants have been taken he will want to know why. The patient may also have been suffering from indigestion for years and taking stomach pills, and it may well be a flare up of the 'indigestion' which has brought him to the hospital on this occasion. He may be taking tablets to control his blood pressure, or other pills which act on the heart, all of which is highly relevant in the present situation. Information on the patient's spare-time interests and exercise habits may also be sought.

Finally the family history is gone into. Are both parents still living? If not what did they die from and at what age? Are there any brothers and sisters, if so are they all well? If any have died, what from and at what age? Is there a family history of any disease such as diabetes, and so on?

As seen, a medical history can cover a great deal of ground and reveal an enormous amount of information, not only on the present problem but also on many of the complicated ramifications that go to make up any one life. And any part of this history may of course be sought in greater detail if it is thought that it may hold a clue towards a firm diagnosis. Such a history may also uncover other problems which require treatment, and any disease process found in its early stages is simpler to treat than one in an advanced stage.

## Physical examination

Provided that the patient is in good condition and not in a state of shock, he will be given a thorough and detailed physical examination.

First the general size and condition of the patient is

noted, with particular reference to the risk factor of obesity. Then the hands – a very useful source of information – are examined: the type of hands, their colour, the condition and shape of the nails. These can provide possible clues to anaemia, a low content of red cells in the blood, and even some types of disease of the heart valves can be picked up by observing the colour of the skin under the nails.

Then the pulse must be taken – obviously one of the most basic and important parts of any examination. It is not sufficient just to record the rate. The rhythm, the character of the pulse, whether weak and thready or banging against the examining fingers, all has to be registered. Here again, clues can be confirmed into facts by this simple procedure.

Next the blood pressure is recorded (for a reminder as to how this is done, see page 23). Blood pressure is clearly of great importance. It may often be found to be raised totally unbeknown to the patient, and this is an important risk factor. In a state of shock the blood pressure falls, sometimes to quite remarkably low levels, which can starve the body of the necessary amount of blood, in which case drugs can be given to correct this.

As the examination proceeds, the neck is closely observed. There are some huge blood vessels in the neck. (Just picture some of the 'muscle men' on television: as they grunt and groan with whatever feats of exertion they are performing, they go red in the face and giant vessels project on the sides of their necks.) It is these neck veins which are observed. They can become engorged, and may even have a pulse transmitted up from the heart if it is under considerable strain and is beginning to 'fail'. Again this may have to be corrected with medication.

Next a close inspection of the eyes is made. Merely looking at the eyes may reveal yellow deposits (*xanthalasma*) in the eyelids. This is suggestive of a raised level of lipids and cholesterol in the blood – another potent risk factor. The lower eyelid when pulled down can reveal whether the patient is anaemic – if the vessels here are pale, this is highly likely. By looking into the eye through an opthalmoscope – a complicated instrument containing a series of lenses – the vessels on the back of the eyeball can be seen clearly. This gives a good indication as to the general condition of the vessels in the rest of the body.

So, before even getting as far as the chest, a considerable amount of information has been sought and possibly found. Several of the risk factors may also have been confirmed. Nicotine on the fingers of a grossly overweight person with elevated blood pressure and xanthalasma – well, he has been asking for it hasn't he?

Now to the chest. The first thing the doctor will do is just look. He may see that the heart is enlarged and heaving, showing it to be working under severe strain. Or there may be virtually no movement of breathing from the chest, the shape of the chest being like a barrel. This is suggestive of a condition called emphysema (see page 21) which is the result of a cough associated with chronic bronchitis, most frequently found in heavy smokers. A variety of problems involving both the heart and lung systems may be found merely by looking. The chest is then 'palpated', that is, felt with the hands. The size of the heart and its movements – or lack of – are confirmed, the character of the heart-beat is defined. This is done by finding the 'apex beat'. In the normal heart there is a tapping on the ribs as the heart beats; the position in which this is felt is noted. If the heart has been under constant strain for a variety of reasons, it may increase in size: there are fairly narrowly defined limits which are acceptable as far as heart size is concerned. If there is a leaking valve or a hole in the heart – that is a gap in the walls dividing the heart chambers – eddies are sometimes set up with the abnormal flow of blood and this can be felt as a 'thrill', exactly like a cat purring.

You will probably have noticed doctors tapping one finger on to the finger of the other hand when examining the chest. This is called 'percussion', and the principle was first discovered in wine cellars. By tapping the barrels they could tell when wine was present by the dull percussion note, and if the barrel was half empty the note above the wine level would be resonant. In just the same way the heart size can be confirmed, as the note there is dull in comparison with the resonant air-filled lungs.

As can be seen, even before the doctor takes up the stethoscope he has already found an enormous amount of information. Each valve has a specific area of the chest where it can be heard, so, by listening to the heart, he can detect any peculiarities – for example, blood flowing through an abnormal valve will make a noise known as a murmur. In heart attacks extra heart sounds can sometimes be heard, or more commonly a disturbance of rhythm which sounds very similar to a horse galloping, the 'gallop rhythm'. This virtually confirms the diagnosis. Sometimes the envelopes of the heart, that is the skin surrounding the heart, become inflamed. This gives yet another noise called a 'rub'.

Movement of air in and out of the lungs can be heard as a clear rise and fall in healthy breathing. If fluid is present in conjunction with heart disease, a crackling noise at the back or bottom of the lungs will be detected.

When the heart and circulatory system have been examined, the ankles will be inspected to discover whether they are swollen and also whether the pulses can be felt. As at the wrists, the arteries at the ankles come close to the skin and should easily be felt there. In hardening of the arteries the pulses of the feet may be absent.

A full physical examination would include the alimentary system – mouth and abdominal contents – the central nervous system and the glandular system, but in the intensive care unit particular attention will be directed at the chest and its contents. If the diagnosis is not clear the abdomen also will come in for close scrutiny, as conditions of the stomach such as ulcers, hiatus hernias or even gall bladder disease can be the cause of the pain which led to admission.

One of the things that puzzles many patients in hospital is why so much blood is taken, sometimes two or three times a day. Is there some vast hungry machine that needs it to survive? The investigation of blood is in fact one of the most important branches of modern medicine. Although it would seem reasonable to assume that one lot of blood would be enough, this is not always the case, and particularly in suspected heart attacks. So why all the blood? The mechanics of a heart attack have been dealt with previously in some detail (page 45), but in brief there is an obstruction in a vessel supplying the heart muscle, which cuts off the food supply and therefore causes the heart muscle to change and begin to die. As this process occurs the muscle releases chemicals called *enzymes* into the bloodstream. These are complicated substances with even more complicated names which it is not necessary to mention: the relevant point is that some enzymes can be discovered in the blood within six hours of the event, while others do not appear until forty-eight hours later, by which time the early ones may be returning to accepted normal levels. Consequently the process and progress of the injury to the heart muscle can be monitored by taking several samples of blood. This can help to define the amount of damage to the heart muscle and assess how the body is coping with the process of repair.

It is not only the heart enzymes which are monitored, although these are the most important; the blood cholesterol and lipid levels will also be analysed. As these may show a falsely low level immediately after a heart attack, the blood is best taken after a fourteen hour fast. So if the white-coated people armed with needles and syringes seem to be coming with monotonous regularity, it is for a very good reason.

Next comes the electrocardiogram (for an explanation of how this works, see page 76). As with the changes that occur within the blood, so with those found on the electrocardiogram, and a series of readings will need to be taken. When a heart attack occurs the electrical activity in that area of muscle ceases. This is called a 'dead electrical window', and may not be apparent for some hours, even up to forty-eight in some cases. So the series of ECGs will show the extent and the site of the damage and whether the healing process is beginning. The heart attack will cause a scar on the heart muscle; as this scar forms and the heart repairs itself, the electrical activity changes are shown over a series of electrocardiograms. Sometimes these changes will appear on the ECG for the rest of the patient's life.

There has been no mention so far of any treatment, and in the case of an uncomplicated heart attack this may consist purely of pain-relieving medication and observation. But until the diagnosis has been proven one way or another it must be assumed that a heart attack has occurred.

In Britain, the chosen drug for relief of pain and apprehension is heroin. This is given by injection; it is the most effective pain-relieving agent known, but it also produces a state of euphoria and sedation.

The observation of the monitor and regular checking of

the blood pressure will continue for at least forty-eight hours until the diagnosis is confirmed. No heart attack, however mild it may appear, can be trusted: any number of events can happen, and treatment may have to be given immediately to rectify the problem in order that the patient may survive.

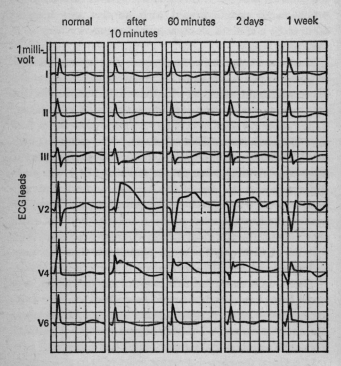

*Changes rapidly take place on the ECG after a heart attack. Several readings are taken in the first few days to find out the site and extent of the attack. The changes shown here have occurred in an anterior heart attack; for a different site the changes will be found in different leads. (For more about leads see pages 79–80.)*

# The complicated
# heart attack

Since the advent of coronary care units there has been a
progressive decline in mortality from acute heart attacks,
providing the patient survives long enough to reach such a
unit. One source quotes a mortality drop to 9 per cent
during the acute stage, in comparison with more than 25
per cent in a similar group of patients cared for in a
general ward. The reason for this decline is better prevention, recognition and management of the acute and highly
dangerous rhythm disturbances that can occur.

As was shown in Chapter 3, the larger the vessel that is
affected, the larger the area of heart muscle involved. So if
one of the major motorways is obstructed, a large area of
muscle will be compromised – as much as 50 per cent of the
left ventricle muscle may be involved. A similar situation
can result if there has been a previous heart attack; the
combination of the two can again result in the involvement
of 40–50 per cent of the heart wall.

It is for these seriously ill people that specialized equipment and staff must be immediately available. Such life-
saving measures as electrical defibrillation (a large
measured electrical shock given to resuscitate a heart
which has stopped or is in a rhythm which if allowed to
continue would cause stoppage) and pacemaking (a small
measured stimulus to regulate heart-beat), together with
positive pressure respirators to assist with breathing, may
be required urgently.

Coronary care units should ideally be small, preferably
sound-proofed, with each bed having its own electrical
supply as well as oxygen and suction units. Each monitor

should be attached to a writing machine so that a permanent record of the progress can be kept for comparison. There should be an alarm set into the monitor so that if the heart goes above or below a pre-set range the staff will be warned immediately. In cases of severe shock, the arterial blood pressure should be monitored by a catheter which is inserted either into the arm or the groin, but otherwise the blood pressure will be frequently checked in the usual way. The chemistry of the blood and its oxygen and carbon dioxide content can be estimated, again on a regular basis if the shock persists.

Whatever equipment is present in these units, it is no substitute for highly trained staff. The equipment is there to help them, but it is only as good as the ability of the staff to recognize the problem for which it has been designed.

## Drug treatment

There is no doubt that the fear and anxiety as well as the pain associated with heart disease can predispose to cardiac arrest, that is the heart stopping. A sleep régime may prove most useful in the case of a particularly anxious person. By regular doses of medication injected into the vein, a carefree state can be induced. This may be lightened during feeding, washing and so on, but can be continued for several days. In a less anxious person, one of several tranquillizers may be helpful.

For the relief of pain, as stated earlier, heroin is the most useful drug and produces fewer of the undesirable side-effects such as nausea and vomiting sometimes associated with more powerful drugs. In some countries heroin is illegal, so an alternative has to be given.

## Oxygen

If a large area of the heart is affected by the attack, the

pump loses its efficiency. This being the case the amount of oxygen in the blood falls and produces a state called *hypoxia* – much the same as that experienced by pilots at high altitudes if cabin pressure fails. Fluid then tends to accumulate at the bottom of the lungs, thereby reducing even further the amount of oxygen that can be 'picked up'. This produces shortness of breath as the oxygen in the blood falls further and the carbon dioxide – the product of cell metabolism – builds up. In an effort to glean more oxygen the heart speeds up, which produces more of a strain on it. This vicious circle is called 'left ventricular failure'. In these circumstances administration of oxygen helps, and each bed in a coronary care unit has oxygen piped to it. In very severe cases it may have to be given by a pump called a ventilator.

## Rhythm problems

Disturbance of the heart's rhythm is one of the main problems in heart attacks. There is, as has been described on page 15, a small fuse box in the heart which is responsible for making it beat regularly, but which is under the control of nerves and chemicals. The nerve that controls the fuse box comes from the brain; if it works overtime as a result of pain, anxiety or fear, the heart rate slows, which may precipitate heart failure followed by bizarre beats occurring over the muscle heart wall called *ectopic activity*. This slow rate, known as *bradycardia*, can be corrected with a drug called atropine given into a vein.

The functioning of the fuse box depends on the impulse being relayed from the atrium through to the major muscular ventricular wall. In a condition called 'heart block' the atria may be receiving the impulse, but this is not picked up by the ventricles. On the electrocardiogram this can easily be seen. In these circumstances, a temporary pacemaker may be used. This is a catheter or narrow tube which is inserted into a vein in either the leg or the arm, and then advanced into the heart. At the tip of this tube there is an electrical output which can give an impulse to the heart at a predetermined rate. There are several different types of pacemakers which are used for temporary treatment, and after a trial period of switching off to see if

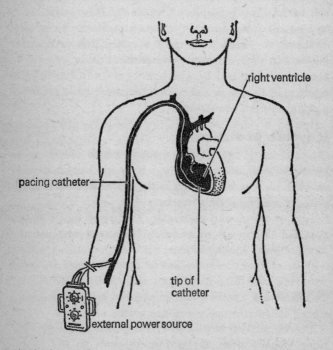

*Artificial pacemakers may be used as a temporary measure, as illustrated, in which case a pacing catheter is attached to a power unit outside the body. If the heart's electrical system fails a permanent pacemaker may be necessary: the power source is then implanted under the skin, or electrodes may be placed directly on to the heart muscle.*

the heart can maintain its beating, they are then removed.

This slowing of the heart rate is not rare – it may be seen in up to 40 per cent of those examined initially – and it is very important that it should be noted as it can alter into highly dangerous rhythms in which the heart loses all semblance of order and the ventricles fibrillate. In this condition the heart muscle flaps in a violent fashion at a rate of about 250–500 per minute, which usually results in the heart stopping (known as *asystole*). Time is very precious in this situation and it must be corrected urgently. Drugs can be given by injection to reduce the tone of the nerve, and the heart rate will then rise.

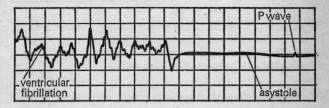

*An electrocardiogram of cardiac arrest. Before the heart stops completely there is a bizarre pattern of electrical activity known as ventricular fibrillation. (This patient was successfully resuscitated, underwent surgery, and is now very well.)*

If the heart rate is unacceptably high or if there are abnormal beats called *ectopics*, then again medication can be given to reduce the rate to acceptable levels. This may either be administered directly into a vein, or if a slow but measured amount of a drug is to be given over some length of time, it will be added to a drip; in this way very careful control of the drug dosage is possible.

After a heart attack the blood pressure may fall, and although a certain drop is acceptable, if it is allowed to fall

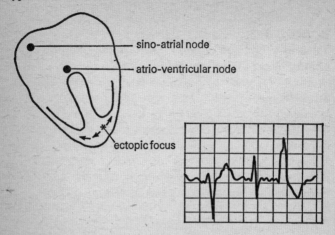

*Ectopic beats. The normal passage of electrical current across the heart is from the sino-atrial node to the atrio-ventricular node to the Bundle of His. Ventricular ectopic beats arise from an impulse other than in the sino-atrial node and produce a bizarre ECG.*

too far permanent damage can result. Here again careful and continued monitoring is important. It may be necessary to give drugs – usually by drip – to stabilize the blood pressure.

When the heart is put under considerable strain, as in a heart attack, the pump – not surprisingly – may lose some of its efficiency. This state, as we have already seen, may require oxygen, but other treatment will be necessary too. This will include medication to help the heart beat more effectively and to rid the circulation of the excess build-up of fluids. This group of drugs is called diuretics, and by assisting in the excretion of fluids from the kidneys they reduce the overload on the circulation, thus breaking the vicious circle. For rapid action, as with most drugs, these can be given directly into veins or administered by a drip.

## Some other drugs

There is a huge selection of drugs that may be used in treating heart conditions, and it is not possible to describe them all here. One or two, however, deserve mention.

*Digitalis* This drug is isolated from the foxglove and has been used in medicine for over a hundred years. Its principal use is in improving the efficiency of the heart contraction, thus enabling the heart to empty more efficiently. It has a direct effect on the conductive tissue – that is the electrical system of the heart – by depressing the sino-atrial and atrio-ventricular nodes, so that the rate of conduction is slowed and more efficient. This remarkable drug has several other applications as well, but in heart failure and rhythm disturbances it has dramatic improving effects.

*Beta blockers* At times of any form of emotional stress – fear, anger, anxiety – a complex variety of changes takes place in the body. This can release substances such as adrenalin and nor-adrenalin, which increase the tone of the sympathetic nervous system, the system dealing with fight and flight. These changes act on receivers in the heart called *adrenergic receptors* which are subdivided into two groups – alpha and beta. Stimulation of the beta adrenoceptors of the heart causes an increase in the heart rate and contractibility, which in turn increases the demand for oxygen by the heart muscle.

Some twenty years ago the first commercial agent to block these receivers was produced on the assumption that – particularly in coronary artery disease – heart work and oxygen demand would be effectively reduced. Since then there has been an explosion in manufacturing beta blocking agents; it appears that any self-respecting drug company has at least one such preparation on the market. They are undoubtedly a great advance in the treatment of coronary artery disease, but they have not been without their problems. One of the early drugs, probably in fact one of the finest beta blockers produced, unfortunately caused severe side-effects principally involving the eyes and the intestines. Now of course all drugs have to pass very stringent safety tests before they are marketed.

The blocking of the receivers and consequent lowering of the heart rate is not the only function of beta blocking drugs. One of the major problems with heart attacks, mentioned earlier, is the development of irregular rhythms that vary in significance from totally unimportant to impending death. The beta blocking agents are used in both the treatment and prevention of these rhythms. They may be used in the short term within the intensive care unit, or the treatment may be continued – even indefinitely. If the blood pressure is elevated or rhythm disturbances persist, the chances of further heart attacks occurring may be reduced by staying on long-term beta blockers.

*Anti-coagulants* Like so many other aspects of the treatment of heart attacks, the use of anti-coagulants is controversial. Some experts maintain that by administering agents which 'thin' the blood by reducing its ability to clot, the overall death rate following heart attacks can be halved; but carefully controlled trials have in some cases failed to bear this out. So whether or not anti-coagulants are used may depend on the views of the doctor under whose care you find yourself. There are, however, certain conditions in which the benefits of anti-coagulants are undeniable. In such cases heparin, which works very rapidly, is given into a vein or by a drip over a period of forty-eight hours while anti-coagulants in tablet form have time to work. When taking these tablets long term, certain precautions are necessary and the dose may have to be altered from time to time. Regular checks have to be made to see that the blood does not become too thin – if this were to happen, there would be a very real risk of bleeding in the absence of the usual control over the clotting mechanism.

# Cardiac arrest

There is absolutely no point in having a well-equipped intensive care unit with a high nurse-to-patient ratio unless there is also a highly trained medical staff familiar with the various procedures which may be necessary in an emergency. Most general hospitals, whether they have an intensive or coronary care unit or not, do have a 'cardiac arrest team' – a team of doctors permanently on call to attend a cardiac arrest at a moment's notice.

If a patient's heart stops beating anywhere within the hospital, the cardiac arrest team is called. Each member of the team carries a 'bleep', a small radio receiver which makes a noise when he is wanted; it may be a two-way receiver or he may have to contact the switchboard to find the location of the emergency. Each member will know whether he has to collect some equipment or go straight to the problem. Measures such as external heart massage and artificial respiration will be taken to resuscitate the patient while the team is on its way.

If a monitor is not already on the patient, one will be applied when the team arrives; if there is no drip, one will be put up; if the patient is not on oxygen, this will be administered, possibly by a respirator machine. Each member will play his part, very rapidly and without panic. If the heart has stopped, this will show as a straight line across the monitor screen. The monitor will also indicate abnormal heart rhythms, and drugs may be used to try to revert these to a more normal state. If there is in fact a cardiac arrest, this requires defibrillation (see page 65). If the first shock does not restore the heart-beat, it may have to be repeated several times to achieve success, by increasing the current.

The decision as to how long such a team should attempt to resuscitate a patient will depend on several factors: how long the arrest took place before treatment was started, what sort of response is being achieved from the treatment, and so on. If the pupils of the eyes remain fully dilated for fifteen minutes, this is an indication to cease, although the decision may be difficult if the patient is on a respirator machine and receiving heart massage.

Patients who survive a cardiac arrest require careful monitoring for at least forty-eight hours, but will then gradually be treated as routine patients. If a cardiac arrest happens while a patient is in hospital there is rarely any long-term problem, and a return to normal life is quite probable.

# 5 Investigating Coronary Artery Disease

The current investigations for heart disease are of two types: 'invasive' and 'non-invasive'. In the former the data is sought by scanning, using various machines which pick up and record the electrical activity of the heart, or in some cases the sound waves. This information is gained without the use of either drugs or needles; the process is entirely painless and the only thing asked of the patient is cooperation. The invasive techniques may involve the application of drugs, or even small tubes called catheters being put into the heart itself; these will be discussed in some detail in Chapter 6. This chapter examines the current non-invasive techniques.

## The electrocardiogram

The form of investigation most often used in heart disease is the electrocardiogram (ECG), and most general practitioners have one. When an ECG is about to be performed, the patient is asked to lie down and relax; this is because all muscles when contracting produce an electrical activity, so in order that only the heart activity is recorded, total relaxation is essential. Just ignore all the wires coming out of the machine – they are there to receive *your* electricity, not to put 2000 volts into *you*.

As long ago as 1887 it was discovered that the electrical current produced by the contraction of the heart muscle could be recorded by means of an instrument called a galvanometer. This principle is used today in clinical electrocardiography: a recording galvanometer is connected to a high gain amplifier which measures the potential differences in current between two chosen points on the patient; as these differences are very small – about 1 millivolt – amplification is obtained by transducers. By convention a 1 millivolt potential difference moves the needle 1 centimetre; a positive potential causes an upward deflection, and vice versa.

Although the heart has four chambers, from an electrical point of view it can be thought of as having only two, because both the atria contract together and both the ventricles likewise; also, as the atria are small they produce only a small deflection – the large deflection comes from the ventricles.

Each mound or line on the ECG is given a letter (the code is international): the P wave is the name given to the contraction of the atrium, the QRS complex is the contraction of the ventricles, and the T wave is the return of the ventricle to the resting state.

The electrical discharge for each beat starts in a small area in the right atrium – the sino-atrial node (S.A. node). This spreads to the next specialized area of nerves in the atrium, the A.V. node (atrio-ventricular), then by very rapid depolarization – first by a single pathway at what is known as the Bundle of His, then into two separate bundles. Once the switch is triggered at the top, the wave of depolarization spreads across the whole heart; it is this change that is recorded by the ECG machine.

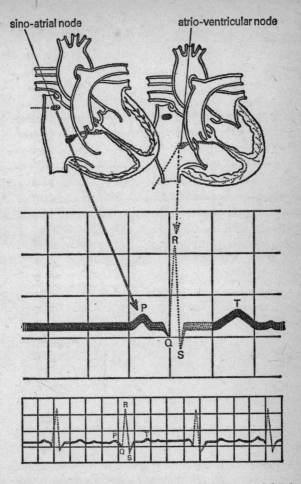

*The electrocardiogram. The P wave represents the discharge of electrical energy from the sino-atrial node which fans across the atria. The QRS segment reflects the progression of the current through the ventricles via the atrio-ventricular node. The T wave is the recharging of the ventricles.*

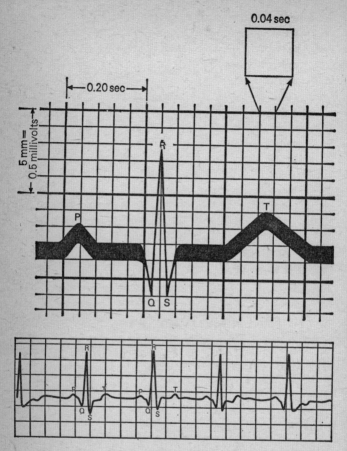

In an electrocardiogram the graph paper measures both time and voltage.
One small square represents horizontally 4/100 of a second, a large
square therefore 1/5 of a second. On the vertical plane 5 millimetres
equals 0.5 millivolts of electricity. The heart rate is calculated by
counting the squares between each R wave and dividing them into 300.
The P wave is the electrical current across the atrium, the QRS across
the ventricles.

In order that the information picked up should be accurately recorded, all ECG machines run at a standard rate: the paper comes out at the same speed, and is divided into graph-like squares which not only give the magnitude of the deflection but also represent time, i.e. five large squares equals one second, one large square 0.2 seconds.

Once you are lying down and have been encouraged to relax, a spider's web of wires will be attached to your body: one to each arm, one to each leg, and then six more across the chest. (You may feel rather like the Bionic Man, but as already said, it is all absolutely painless.) Each of these leads gives a single reading so that the heart can be looked at from several directions. The limb leads look at the heart in a vertical plane – from the sides or from the feet – so leads I, II and aVL look at the left lateral surface of the heart. Leads III and aVF look at the lower surface, and lead aVR at the atria. The chest or V leads are fixed to the

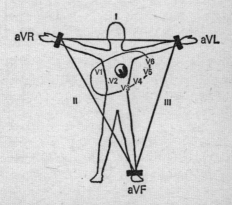

*In order that the heart may be viewed in both planes, several leads have to be used. The limb leads (aVR, aVL, aVF and I-III) look at the heart in the vertical plane, the chest leads (V1–V6) look directly down on the heart.*

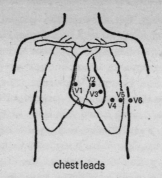

chest leads

*The electrical fields of the electrocardiogram. There are six leads attached to the chest; the positioning of these leads, described in the text below, is of the utmost importance as each looks down on specific areas of the heart.*

chest with suction cups and these leads look directly at the heart in the horizontal plan, that is from the front. V1 and V2 look at the right ventricle, V3 and V4 the septum between the ventricles and the front wall of the left ventricle. V5 and V6 look at the front and side walls of the left ventricle.

With each beat the heart changes its electrical potential. This change is picked up by the electrocardiogram, and depending on which site is being 'looked at' the ECG line is converted to a positive upward deflection or a negative downward one.

From this brief description of the basic principles of electrocardiography you will see that it is an invaluable diagnostic tool in the investigation of rhythm changes, conduction abnormalities, changes of the ventricle, and of course heart attacks. In the latter not only does it tell the physician what part of the heart is involved, it is also of great use in observing the changes that take place as the muscle begins to heal.

# Exercise or stress tests

The very name of this investigation may be enough to provoke a relapse in some people, but there is really no need to be apprehensive about the procedure at all.

When you buy a car or other piece of machinery, you will want to know not only what it looks like, but how it has performed in test conditions at maximum output. Many of the mechanical problems are only obvious at the higher levels of output, and this is the theory behind exercise testing the heart: an electrocardiogram is of great assistance but it only records the state of the resting heart – exercise testing is a method of investigating hearts under stress through exercise.

It has been known for some time that exercise in patients with coronary artery disease produces a change in the ST segment of the electrocardiogram. As far back as 1918 a depression of this segment was noted in an attack of angina, and ten years later it was reported that this also occurred with exercise. Changes and advances since then have produced an interesting history of exercise testing, but with improved technology and the advent of computers, analysis is becoming more sophisticated and accurate in the investigation of early coronary heart disease.

The early exercise testing was performed simply by the patient treading on and off a step, an ECG being taken immediately after the exercise. This step-test is still popular in some centres, but the two methods now widely used are either the static cycle (ergometer) or the treadmill. The latter sounds like some medieval penal exercise, but in fact it is an accurate piece of scientific equipment consisting of a belt on which one walks – usually the gradient of this can be raised and lowered and the speed altered.

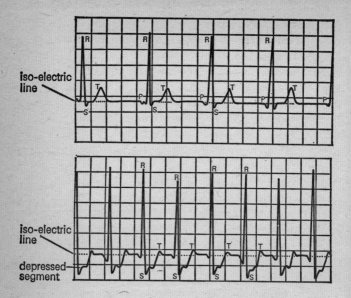

*ECG changes during an exercise test. The top trace was taken at rest: the heart rate is 75 beats per minute and the ST segment is on the iso-electric line. The bottom trace shows a heart rate of 150 and a completely changed wave pattern. The ST segment has sagged below the iso-electric line, indicating severe coronary heart disease.*

Before the test itself is performed, it is important that a resting ECG is taken first. This is to make sure that there are no changes going on which would make the test a danger; if the heart is to be asked to work as hard as it can, then every precaution must be taken that it is safe for it to do so. This being the case, electrodes are placed on the chest; these can either be attached to a monitor by a direct lead, or to a small radio transmitter carried on a belt which then transmits the heart to a receiver (radio-telemetry). The latter has the advantage of there being no cumbersome wires. (Incidentally this is a useful gadget in that it may have a radio range of several hundred yards, and research into stress suffered by racing drivers, for example, has been done using radio-telemetry.)

My personal choice involves the use of direct wire 12-lead ECG and the treadmill. Cooperation between patient and doctor is vital. All symptoms felt during the test must be reported, such as chest pain, shortness of breath and so on. The treadmill starts at a slow rate and low gradient – it may take a minute or two to gain the skill required in using it, but rarely any longer. The monitor is carefully observed, and the test progresses with increases in both rate and gradient after a predetermined time; this has the advantage of setting a precedent so that, should the test have to be repeated, the same procedure is used and an accurate comparison can be made. This is particularly useful in assessing the progress of drug treatment or surgery.

The exercise test will continue until either the patient says he can't go on – although often with some encouragement or reassurance he may be persuaded to do so for a little longer – or the physician decides, for a variety of reasons, to stop it. The physician may have set a 'target heart rate', that is, a rate which he considers would give him all the information he wants; or there may be changes on the screen, or changes in the blood pressure which will have been taken frequently during the test. Immediately after the exercise the patient either lies or sits relaxing while the readings continue, and a repeat resting ECG may be taken.

A recent and more sophisticated version of this exercise test, which it is thought will give a more accurate diagnosis as to which part of the heart is damaged, is still in its infancy as a research programme. It is called 'precordial mapping', and the basic idea is the same as for the exercise

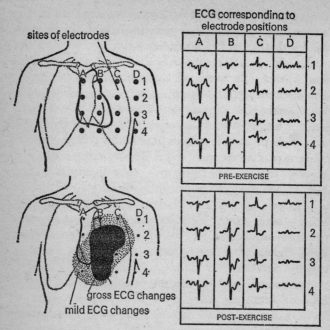

*Precordial mapping. This technique 'maps' the diseased area of the heart. The top diagram shows the position of the electrodes and the corresponding ECG. Below, the diseased area is mapped out from the ECG changes shown.*

test mentioned, but instead of only one or two electrodes being used, a total of sixteen leads are attached to the chest so that a grid is produced. It is thought that the readings obtained will show not only whether the heart is under some strain, but the actual area of the strain.

## The purpose of exercise testing

**1.** *Screening.* It is still widely believed that significant coronary artery disease produces angina, and that a good diagnostic physician can elicit evidence of coronary disease during a full physical work-out by questioning the patient about his chest pain. But it has also been shown quite clearly that the test can pick up heart disease which has previously gone unrecognized. Two trials reported from Long Beach, California, showed that of 284 executives who were thought to be normal, 11 per cent were found to have positive tests (i.e. abnormal exercise ECGs) with no chest pains; in another trial of 1000 people, only 37 per cent with positive tests were suffering from chest pain. There are doctors who would dispute the accuracy of exercise testing, but I feel very strongly that anything which leads towards early diagnosis must be worth while.

**2.** *Chest pain of unknown origin.* The diagnosis of ischaemic heart disease poses little problem if there is the classic history of angina (see page 39). But so often there is doubt: the pain may be angina; there again, it may be of no cardiac significance, and it is clearly wrong to label a patient as suffering from heart disease if there is any doubt. Exercise testing can frequently give the answer.

**3.** *Evaluation of treatment.* Exercise testing is a repeatable investigation and is therefore a useful way of assessing the effectiveness of treatment. The pulse rate can be plotted against the amount of exercise taken – in this way, the improvement achieved with drug treatment and surgery can also be recorded, so that an accurate comparison may be made. One way to plot this is demonstrated in the diagram on page 86. The vertical column is the pulse rate; the horizontal line is the work load. As the heart's efficiency improves, the pulse rate is seen to be lower for the same amount of work – or to achieve the same pulse rate as before, a greater amount of exercise has to be taken.

**4.** *Prescribing exercise.* Finding out just what can be achieved by these tests gives a very useful yardstick as to exercise capabilities, in terms both of recreation and of occupation.

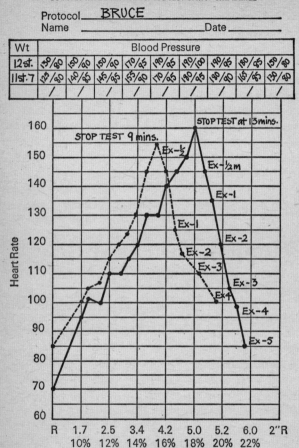

Protocol __BRUCE__

Name _____ Date _____

| Wt | Blood Pressure | | | | | | | | |
|---|---|---|---|---|---|---|---|---|---|
| 12 st. | 130/60 | 150/60 | 150/60 | 170/65 | 190/65 | 190/100 | 190/85 | 180/85 | 130/80 |
| 11 st. 7 | 125/60 | 140/65 | 145/65 | 155/60 | 170/65 | 190/95 | 190/90 | 165/85 | 120/80 |
|  | / | / | / | / | / | / | / | / | / |

Plotting heart rate against work load in exercise testing; this chart is
used for a test performed on the treadmill. The heart rate achieved each
minute is plotted against the speed and gradient of the treadmill. The
rate of recovery is recorded after exercise, and blood pressure is noted
both during and after exercise. This test is accurate and repeatable, and
is consequently very useful in monitoring drug and surgical treatment.

**5.** *Investigation of heart rhythm disturbances.* One of the most useful outcomes of exercise testing is to find out the effect of increases in the heart rate on any abnormal rate or rhythm which has been discovered either by examination or by a resting electrocardiogram. The changes found at exercise are of very great significance, and treatment will depend on the results found.

As I have already pointed out, it is often only after someone has actually suffered a heart attack that he is sufficiently motivated to follow medical advice on giving up smoking, losing weight, changing his diet and lifestyle, and so on. This falls into the category of secondary prevention; exercise testing can provide a strong motivation for following such advice at a stage when prevention is still possible.

# Twenty-four hour tape monitoring

All of us today are familiar with gramophone records, and most of with the more recent invention of tape-recorders and cassettes. In the field of cardiology this marvel of modern electronics has been adapted to join the widening range of non-invasive investigation techniques available.

When a person who has been experiencing some discomfort in the chest presents himself to the doctor, he may be feeling really very well at the time. He then tries to explain in detail the episodes of palpitations or racing heart, which may last for several hours before they pass off. He may complain of chest pains associated with the palpitations, but they may only occur infrequently. In order to get a clearer picture of what is happening, the doctor may decide to use a twenty-four hour ambulatory tape.

This involves the patient carrying with him on a belt around his waist a small tape-recorder which runs at a slow speed for twenty-four hours. The recorder is attached by electrodes to the chest in a manner similar to that for exercise testing, and firmly secured. This box of tricks is not heavy and is no hindrance to the person carrying out his normal activities. Once the electrodes have been placed on the chest – and to get good results this must be done with great care – the machine starts to record. Before being sent off, all patients are given an 'event diary'. Whenever the palpitation, pain or any other symptom is felt the time is noted in the diary, as is the activity which is being undertaken at that time. Any other event which may change the heart's activity (such as speech-making, arguments, sexual intercourse, and so on) is also noted, to see just what is happening to the heart.

It can be seen that this instrument is a very useful piece of research equipment, not only in investigating people with heart problems, but also in finding out what happens to normal hearts when subjected to various stimuli, either physical or psychological. Racing-car drivers, airline pilots, parachutists and public speakers have all been investigated in this manner – often with fascinating and unexpected results.

Twenty-four hour tape monitoring gives a much more realistic picture than laboratory experiments in artificial conditions. So much of the early research on sexual intercourse, for example, was performed in laboratories, with slightly suspect volunteers, that it was thought the heart response reached levels close to the limit of its capabilities. This idea changed rapidly, however, when normal married couples were investigated in their home environment, and it has now been found that sex is not the potentially lethal pastime it was once thought to be.

After the recorder has been worn for a complete day, the tape is taken off and is fed into a machine, which converts the tape-recorder to an ECG pattern on a screen. (The biggest disadvantage of this investigation is the very high cost of this machine.) Interpretation of the tapes is a highly skilled procedure. The record is 'edited' and samples taken, either of events detailed in the diary (the interpretation machine is calibrated with the time of the tape recording), or of sections showing up abnormalities on the screen as the tape runs. The final analysis is interpreted by a heart specialist familiar with this technique.

Twenty-four hour monitoring is particularly useful when investigating people who are thought to have some abnormality of the heart rhythm and palpitations. It is important to know, if this is suspected, what type of rhythm is occurring and from where in the fuse box and electrical system of the heart the problem is arising. Once this has been ascertained, the appropriate treatment can be given. This type of monitoring is not the sole answer, and like all such procedures it can give false positive and false negative information, but with these reservations it is still an important part of the heart specialist's armoury.

# Echo-cardiography

The echo-cardiogram is a sophisticated piece of machinery developed along the lines of asdic and sonar, the echo-locating devices so crucial during the Second World War in looking for submarines.

This is not the place to go into the physics of acoustic resistance, frequency of oscillations, and so on; it is enough to say that there exists a device called a transducer which converts one type of energy into another, in this case an electrical one into an acoustic one and vice versa. The main echoes received from the heart are at the blood interspaces in the muscle, and there are almost none at all from a blood-filled vessel.

The echoes are reflected back to the transducer and converted into an electrical impulse, and a visual display is then produced on the fluorescent screen of an oscilloscope. There are various types of display which are constantly being improved, and perhaps the combined use of ultrasonics and laser beams will one day provide a three-dimensional cross section of a pulsating heart.

# Radio-active scanning

In a few specialized units in Britain there is another method of investigation which is extremely useful. This is the use of a small amount of radio-active isotope material injected into a vein. Healthy heart muscle will absorb a certain amount of the isotope – thalium is the most common in use – whereas damaged muscle will absorb a different amount. The amount of radio-activity given off, which is very small, can be registered on a photographic film. By showing the difference between a healthy and a damaged heart muscle, the film can reveal what area of the heart is involved and how it behaves during both exercise and rest.

This investigation is still in the early stages, but it has very exciting prospects for the future. It is safe and – apart from the injection into the vein, which will only upset the greatest cowards among us – completely painless. As the technique develops it may eventually supersede the investigation involving cardiac catheterization.

# 6 Cardiac Surgery – Why?

'What can be done if my angina gets worse in spite of the tablets?' 'Is there any place for surgery after heart attacks?' 'What sort of surgery could I have and how does it work?'

These are all very reasonable questions, but as with virtually every facet of this subject they will provoke considerable differences of opinion in the medical profession. Great advances have been made in heart surgery over the past decade; heart transplantation – in particular the first such operation by Dr Christian Barnard in the 1960s – has made headlines in the world press, although this is a highly specialized subject beyond the scope of this book.

The surgery currently performed for ischaemic heart disease is known as coronary artery by-pass grafting. There is a major difference of opinion on opposite sides of the Atlantic about surgery in general and coronary artery by-pass grafting in particular. In America this operation is relatively common – 100,000 were performed there in one year – while in Britain only the major hospitals sport the necessary highly specialized team of surgeons, technicians, nursing staff and equipment.

The non-invasive methods of investigation described in the last chapter provide a great deal of information, sometimes – as for instance when the heart requires valvular surgery – enough to justify an operation without any further investigation. But in coronary disease involving the blood supply of the heart, non-invasive techniques will show only that some vessels are involved; they will not show which vessel, how much of it is affected, or how many others are in trouble. To make an accurate diagnosis, an angiogram (or coronary arteriogram or coronary catheterization) will have to be done. This is what is meant by an invasive technique, involving the injection of a substance into the heart circulation; the result is watched on an X-ray screen.

# Angiograms

## What is an angiogram?

X-ray examinations are commonplace in medicine today. They were discovered by Wilhelm Röntgen, a German, in 1895 and it was not long before doctors were experimenting with potential clinical applications – broken bones were first. In the following year, two German scientists injected a substance into the blood vessels of an amputated hand and demonstrated for the first time the possibility of outlining the blood vessels: the substance injected is not penetrated by the X-rays and is known as radio-opaque. The search was on to find a substance that could be injected into a living person without ill-effects, and in the early 1920s first two French scientists with a mixture of oil and iodine, then two German scientists with a bromide solution, injected arteries to show the arterial tree, and later veins in the same way. In 1924 an American surgeon injected sodium iodide into the leg and showed that it was possible to observe the arterial blood supply and to judge whether operation was necessary in the case of disease of the arteries. So began the clinical application of arteriography.

The first problem was to perfect a safe solution for injection: the ideal solution had to provide accurate visualization without side-effects, and research continued until the various materials used today were found. The next hurdle was to develop a technique which would not only outline all the vessels of the heart, but record the action of the heart as it was beating. Taking a straight X-ray of the heart produces a picture of one instant only, and in order to detect abnormalities of blood flow, disease or malformation, a combination of X-ray and cine-film known as cineangiography was developed. A high-speed film of 15–60 frames a second or a serial film of 6–12 frames a second is used, the high-speed one being particularly useful for detecting abnormalities of blood flow in valvular disease, holes in the heart and coronary artery disease. The 35mm film used can be projected and the action of the heart observed, and the film can be stopped at any frame so that the outline of the vessels may be observed for any abnormality.

There are a number of indications for cardiac catheterization – problems in the right side of the heart, investigation of the arteries going to the lungs, congenital heart disease, trouble in the valves of the heart – but we are concerned here with the investigation of the coronary arteries.

## How is it done?

As its name implies, an invasive technique involves insertion of instruments and solutions into the body, so the investigation is carried out in hospital. A large amount of equipment is necessary, not only the X-ray machine and a battery of monitoring screens but, as in any other branch of surgery, the back-up facilities for any emergency.

Angiograms are usually done under a local anaesthetic and the patient will be fully conscious; he will however have an injection beforehand – similar to that given before any operation – to allay any very natural anxiety. After the injection, he will be taken to the catheter laboratory and put on to an operating table.

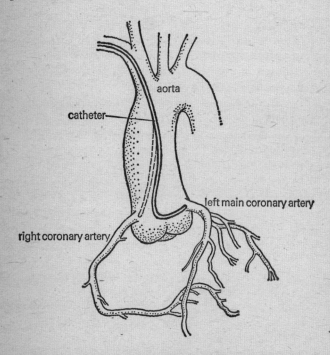

*Coronary arteriography. The catheter is fed into the aorta from an artery in the arm or leg; its position is followed on an X-ray screen and it is inserted into the opening of each coronary artery.*

The catheter has to be fed into the left side of the heart (the left side is used as it is here that the aorta leaves the heart and the coronary arteries branch off), through an artery, usually the brachial artery. A small injection of local anaesthetic, similar to a local dental anaesthetic, is injected into the arm so that no pain at all will be felt at the incision to expose the artery – perhaps a slight pulling sensation may be experienced as the artery is exposed, but this is more uncomfortable than painful.

A wide-bore needle is inserted into the artery through which is passed a thin-walled, flexible tube; this is threaded on a guideline up through the artery. The process can be watched on a large screen that looks like a television but is in fact an X-ray image intensifier – much like those that used to be in shoe shops, in which you could see your toes in the shoes you were about to buy. The heart can be seen beating, and soon the tip of the catheter appears as a thin dark line moving slowly up towards the heart. Some people find this fascinating, others don't want to know, but either way it is not a painful experience.

The catheter is radio-opaque so that the operator can see where it is in relation to the heart; it is made of special nylon or Teflon, and may have a hole at the end or, more usually in coronary artery investigation, holes at the side, or both. Once the catheter is near the heart, a solution is flushed through it to prevent the blood clotting, then a small amount of the dye is injected, a sort of test dose to make sure that there will be no adverse reaction to the dye. With the catheter safely inserted in the left side of the heart, the X-ray film will start (this is quite noisy) and the dye will be introduced through the catheter. This is seen immediately on the screen as dark and rapidly moving, and is then very quickly washed away. It gives a sudden feeling of heat which starts in the chest and spreads through the body, a strange rather than painful sensation – not too distressing if one is expecting it – which soon passes.

The catheter tip is now withdrawn from the heart and passed into the opening of the right-sided coronary artery, and another injection of the dye is made and filmed from the front and the side so that the whole length of the artery may be clearly seen. The dye can be seen along the whole course of the vessels, and one patient described it as if 'a light shone inside my heart' – indeed it does look as though a torch is displaying the arterial tree. After investigation of the right artery has been completed, the catheter is introduced into the left, larger coronary; again several views are taken and any shortcoming in one view will be clarified in the other. Once more, a film is made of the whole course of the dye and a permanent record made which can be stopped at any point to clarify the condition of the artery.

During the investigation various other observations are made – a series of pressures within the heart and the electrocardiogram are recorded, for example. When all the data is collected, the catheter is withdrawn, the artery closed, the skin incision stitched and a small dressing applied. There should be no further discomfort, but a rest in bed is necessary to ensure there are no delayed reactions to the dye. The risk of complications is as low as 0.1 per cent, but as in all medicine, it cannot be eliminated entirely.

## How are the results interpreted?

When the film has been developed it is projected on to a screen and analysed by the cardiologists. The outline of the arteries is carefully observed to see if there is any blockage or restriction of flow along the vessel. Particularly important is the degree of an obstructive process, which may vary from slight narrowing to a complete obstruction of the vessel: surprisingly it is not until there is a 50 per cent narrowing of the vessel that the blood flow decreases significantly. The extent and pattern of the blockage is important – in many patients the area affected tends to be localized, with a fairly normal healthy artery beyond the obstruction. If this is so, then regardless of how severe or extensive the obstruction, surgery can be performed, providing there is sufficient normal arterial tree beyond it and the heart muscle wall has not been too severely affected.

It will help to visualize the anatomy of the artery tree. You may remember that there are two main vessels: the right and the larger left coronary arteries. The left has a main trunk dividing into two branches, (1) the anterior descending, going down over the front of the heart, and (2) the circumflex, passing behind it. In the diagram below you can see where these vessels are most often obstructed. The

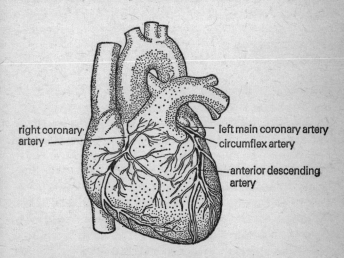

*Some sites of blockages of the coronary artery circulaion. Any one or all three of these major vessels may be affected.*

terms single, double and triple vessel disease are used, according to the number of vessels involved.

A recent advance which adds to the accuracy of this test is the injection of a radio-active substance into the coronary arteries. This emits gamma rays, and with the use of a gamma camera and computer, the area of the starved heart muscle can be plotted.

The coronary angiogram is the final investigation that the cardiologist has at his disposal. Together with the results of all the other tests, he now has an enormous amount of information to help him decide upon treatment. If, despite the medical treatment already discussed, the patient's quality of life remains poor – because of severe pain or discomfort brought on by low levels of exercise, emotion, food, or any of the precipitating factors already mentioned – the problem will have to go before the cardiac surgeon.

# Surgery

### By-pass grafting

The most common operation today, coronary artery by-pass grafting, will be undertaken only after joint consultation between the physician and the heart surgeon, who will take into account the results of all the investigations – the exercise test and coronary angiogram in particular. Their main consideration will be the extent to which the patient's life is affected by angina; there is no doubt that the results of a severely handicapped patient undergoing surgery can be miraculous – described by one as 'a rebirth'.

Whether surgery also increases life expectancy is still not known, although comparison groups of several thousands of people are at present being studied. If there is a blockage of the left main branch of the coronary artery system, before it divides into the circumflex and anterior descending arteries, it appears that surgery to this vessel can not only improve the quality of life but also increase longevity. There is also some evidence that the same may apply in the case of two or three of the main vessels being blocked.

## How is it done?

The operation is of course performed under a general anaesthetic, and a heart–lung machine is used to support the patient during the actual by-pass grafting. The procedure is the same whether one, two or three grafts are to be inserted. The blockages already seen on the angiogram are identified at operation and a vein is stitched in place in front of the blockage and beyond it, thus creating a diversion – or by-pass – so that the blood can flow freely to the muscle supplied by that vessel. It is the starving of the muscle of oxygen which causes angina, so enabling more oxygen to get to the muscle by this by-passing of the narrowed or blocked vessel should greatly reduce the pain and probably get rid of it altogether.

There is a large vein in the leg called the long saphenous vein which goes from the inside of the ankle right up to the groin (it is this vessel which, if it loses its efficiency and becomes varicose, produces those lumpy legs associated with varicose veins). The body can function perfectly well without this vein, so this is the one used to form the by-pass. As in all veins there are small flap valves on the inside of the vessel, and it must be grafted so that the blood flows in the same direction as it did in the leg. As the tissue comes from the same person there is no likelihood of the heart discarding the newly inserted vessel.

At operation, the heart is exposed by splitting the breastbone along its entire length; as the coronary arteries lie on the surface it is not too difficult to identify them, and with the help of the information supplied by the angiogram the site of the blockage should be found quite quickly. The patient is connected to the heart–lung machine, which temporarily takes over the work of the heart so that surgery can continue without the disturbance of a constantly beating heart. A cut about a quarter of an inch long is then made into the vein to be used for grafting, which is bevelled and trimmed to fit the artery and sewn into place with fine, delicate sutures. Once this is done, the clamp over the aorta is released and blood starts to flow again along the

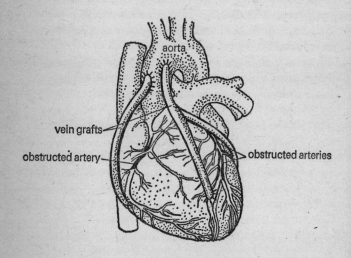

*Coronary artery by-pass graft surgery. The number of grafts inserted depends on how many of the coronary arteries are obstructed; the diagram shows extensive disease of all arteries which have been by-passed. The graft, which is stitched into place, passes directly from the aorta to beyond the obstruction in each artery, thereby increasing the supply of blood to the muscle.*

coronary arteries; within a few seconds the heart will start to beat. Sometimes it has to be stimulated by an electrical shock, but it is quite capable of tolerating a reduced blood flow for 15 minutes while the stitching is being done.

Exactly the same procedure will be used if other vessels are involved, and finally the heart–lung machine will be disconnected and the main incision closed. Post-operative care is given in the intensive care unit, with constant monitoring of pulse, blood pressure and so on, and recovery is usually very rapid.

The results of this operation, in both the short and long term, are usually excellent and the risk is very low – about 2 per cent. There is a relief of symptoms in about 90 per cent of people, 60 per cent with total relief and 30 per cent with considerable improvement. Quality of life is usually enormously improved, and people have frequently returned to a job involving more physical activity than they were capable of previously.

One of the most reliable ways of assessing the benefit of surgery is to perform an exercise test (described on page 81) under standard conditions, using a set protocol which can be repeated. Frequently the indication for stopping the test is increasing chest pain; when the test is performed after the operation there may be no pain at all, and an ability to achieve much greater work-loads than before the operation underlines its success.

## Other operations

There are other operations for clearing blocked arteries. One of these is endarterectomy, in which the blockage in the artery is cleared from the vessel wall. The artery is opened from well above to below the site of the block, and a line of separation found between the plaque and the artery wall; then the plaque is split off the wall – much like peeling an orange – using carbon dioxide gas under pressure, and the vessel is carefully sewn up again. It is a procedure which can only be carried out in the case of a very clearly localized blockage, and is used much less often than by-pass grafting.

Sometimes the scar tissue left in the heart muscle after a heart attack may weaken under the constant pressure of the beating heart; this causes what is known as an aneurysm, a bulge in the wall, just as a worn place in a tyre will bulge if over-inflated. Obviously this makes for inefficient action of the heart muscle – indeed the aneurysm may be working against the beating heart rather than with it, and in this case heart failure will result. So it may be decided to remove this useless section of the heart muscle by surgery. The patient is connected to a heart–lung machine and the 'blow-out' area removed, then the muscle is sutured together and the heart wall restored. The results of this operation are excellent, but again, it will only help some people and these must be selected with great care.

There is a further advance in the treatment of atheroma in coronary disease with the forbidding title of 'percutaneous transluminal angioplasty'. This is an attempt to reduce the extent of the procedure in treating the plaques of atheroma in the vessels, and it is still in the experimental stage. The blockage in one of the coronary vessels having first been identified by the standard methods already described, a catheter is then fed up into the heart in much the same way as for the coronary angiogram. Special guide wires are used to direct the catheter into the right or left coronary artery, and a contrast medium is used to trace its route on a TV screen. When the tip of the catheter, which contains a small balloon, reaches the narrowed or blocked part of the vessel the balloon is inflated by a very accurately controlled pump; this crushes the plaque of fatty tissue on the wall of the vessel, thus reducing the blockage, improving the potency of the vessel and allowing a better blood flow without having to resort to the major surgery of by-pass grafting.

Not everyone with coronary artery disease is suitable for this treatment and there is a fairly rigorous selection procedure: the patient should be under 50 years of age, should not have had symptoms – such as angina – for more than 9 months, and most important of all should have a well-defined blockage which is not occluding the whole vessel (this would prevent the tip of the catheter from getting through). But results so far are very encouraging, and the day may come when it supersedes much of the surgery now being carried out.

## To operate or not

There are times when a patient faces a considerable dilemma caused by the difference of opinion about cardiac surgery on opposite sides of the Atlantic. The story of a patient of mine illustrates the point. This man is a senior executive in a multi-national company based in America. He had a heart attack in London and came to me for a rehabilitation course; the damage to his heart had resulted in a small aneurysm in the ventricle which could be clearly identified on his ECG and was confirmed at exercise test. He was – and is – however an extremely strong man and outstandingly fit, pain-free and with no physical limitations on his life at all. When he returned to the United States, he was reviewed by the Company doctors there and strongly advised to have surgery, a course of action which had been discussed and discarded by his doctors in London. By the time he returned to England he was totally confused: opinion in America made it clear that surgery was the obvious answer, while the English cardiologists, though acknowledging the presence of an aneurysm, felt that his quality of life and general fitness made it unnecessary for him to undergo an operation. He took the advice of the latter and is now very well, with no pain in his chest at any time.

This tale does not prove one side right and the other wrong, but it does highlight the difficulty for the patient of conflicting medical attitudes. On whichever side of the Atlantic, members of the profession make their decisions after considerable thought and care and in the light of their experience. Whether this is a conservative medical approach or a more radical surgical one may well depend on local factors such as facilities for investigation or the availability of a competent surgeon.

The benefits of surgery will also depend very largely on patient cooperation. There is little point in having grafts put in and then adopting a lifestyle which ignores all the risk factors that brought about the need for surgery in the first place. Every effort must be made to reduce risks: no smoking, regular exercise, reasonable weight levels, low consumption of animal fats and a better organization of life to avoid too much stress. These are cardinal rules, and if they are ignored there is a strong possibility that the grafts will become blocked and the crippling symptoms of angina will reappear.

out imposing a load on the heart, and to start a psychological adjustment (this is the time for the experienced patient mentioned above to begin his work).

2. The patient is out of bed, can walk about and manage a flight of stairs. He may soon leave the hospital – usually a week or 10 days after coming in – but even this short time is enough for him to become dependent on the sanctuary and safety of the hospital. This stage will end when the best possible functional recovery has been made and work has been resumed – or if this is not feasible, then the maximum physical capability has been achieved. The psychological aspects must continue to be dealt with during this time: confidence to cope with the demands and pressures of a full life must be regained.

3. The aim of the third stage is to maintain the maximum physical and psychological levels achieved at the end of the convalescent stage. This will continue for the rest of the patient's life.

Return to work is greatly to be encouraged; it has been shown that – given the appropriate job – it is less harmful to continue working than to prolong inactivity. Loss of self-esteem, to say nothing of financial hardship, can prove disastrous to the patient and his family, although of course the type of job is relevant. At one end of the scale is the self-employed small businessman, whose business loses every day he is away; at the other end of the scale is the man in a very routine job which he possibly hates, in a big company or government department which allows six months' sick leave on full pay. In the first case it may be hard to stop the self-employed man from returning to the very circumstances that helped land him in the coronary care unit in the first place; in the other case, the incentive to get back to work is very low until the sick leave has expired. There are some jobs such as driving trains or flying aeroplanes to which, by law, it is not possible to return; in this case, an alternative and satisfying job in the same organization is the ideal solution.

Only a few years ago, the standard treatment after a heart attack was at least six weeks in hospital followed by a long period of rest at home – at the end of which self-confidence and general morale had probably reached rock bottom. But there is now a great deal of evidence to show that early mobilization does not increase the danger to the patient and that an active programme of physical exercise is really beneficial; indeed patients following this active approach are likely to return to work earlier and in greater numbers than those who have been left to fend for themselves. Early encouragement and guidance, psychologically and physically, must go hand in hand. In one survey 70 per cent of patients who had not received this guidance showed some degree of disability when followed up four years later, but after assessment and treatment as outlined above, a striking improvement was seen both in personal and family morale.

# Physical rehabilitation

In most cases, especially when the heart attack has been a mild and uncomplicated one, the family doctor has an increasingly important part to play in encouraging, guiding and advising his patient on his return from hospital. And as physical training becomes more widely recognized as an important part of rehabilitation, help may be needed from a special unit at a hospital to fulfil this need.

Advice on physical rehabilitation is usually given in one of four ways. On leaving the hospital, in consultation with either the patient's own doctor or the hospital doctor and with the help of a small booklet, specific advice may be offered on exactly how much exercise should be taken and how that exercise should progress through convalescence and afterwards. In the early months graded exercises, under supervision and adapted to individual needs, may be undertaken in a formal exercise programme at a special clinic or hospital outpatient department. Preferably these should be done in small groups, which adds the benefit of mutual encouragement. The third method is a gymnasium-type physical training programme carried out in the laboratory; in these programmes high levels of heart rates are reached under monitor control – the aim is for peak fitness and highly trained specialist staff and equipment are required. The last and least satisfactory method – unfortunately still very common in Britain today – is to leave the patient to his own devices, with advice limited to: 'Just do what you feel like doing'. One of the aims of this book is to show that such advice is no longer acceptable in the light of more modern thinking.

The exercise laboratory is not generally practicable and some doctors would disagree with it anyway; although it is possible to train people who have had heart attacks to very high levels of physical activity, there is an associated risk, albeit a small one. This leaves the first two methods, and it is a combination of these that I shall look at now. Obviously it is unrealistic to keep people in hospital for several weeks after a heart attack just so that they can attend a rehabilitation programme – and anyway, most people want to get home as soon as possible. So the exercise programme can be run as an outpatient clinic, with attendance two or three times a week for some weeks, followed by encouragement and guidance from the family doctor and possibly the use of a small booklet on graduated exercise. Physical training will help the coronary patient to overcome fear and anxiety and long-term inactivity, and to develop self-confidence; often the need for tablets and drugs can be reduced. At the start of the programme, an assessment must be made of fitness potential and, within those limits, up to 90 per cent of those partaking will be able to lead a full and enjoyable life.

Heart attacks can be roughly divided into three categories: *mild and uncomplicated* – no significant complications during the illness and no abnormal symptoms afterwards; *moderate or slightly complicated* – significant but not severe complications during the illness, and abnormal pulse rhythms, enlargement of the heart, angina or shortness of breath in the convalescent period; *severe or complicated* – extreme abnormalities of rhythm, serious enlargement, permanent in the heart muscle, and severe angina and/or shortness of breath at rest.

With these categories in mind, the management of each heart attack should be assessed individually. People in the first group will usually progress uneventfully. Those in the second group can go either way: with positive guidance they will do very well, but left to their own devices there is a chance that they will develop into cardiac neurotics from ignorance and fear rather than from actual disease. Those having suffered a severe heart attack present more of a problem; further tests may have to be done and surgery may be suggested in some cases, but even if the damage is too severe for such treatment, some form of rehabilitation other than exercise will help to restore morale.

## Mobilization programmes

The major risk in the acute stage of a heart attack is a severe abnormality of the beating rhythm developing. This happens most commonly in the first two days – hence the coronary care unit with its television monitoring – but once this period of danger has passed, rehabilitation should begin.

In America, a system of measuring exercise is widely used based on the energy requirements of the body: 1 MET is the basic requirement for sitting still in a chair, and from this basic measurement a table of comparisons has been developed – for example, standing or walking very slowly, $1\frac{1}{2}$ METs, typing or walking at 2 miles an hour, 2–3 METs, bricklaying, golf, pulling a trolley, 3–4 METs, and so on up to 10 METs for shovelling quickly, competitive squash, etc. (See the table of metabolic equivalents, pages 145–7.) Booklets are available giving advice related to these equivalents which have proved very helpful in planning exercise routines and rehabilitation programmes.

## Stages in mobilization

1. Limited limb movements to encourage circulation, breathing exercises, face washing and/or shaving, cleaning teeth, eating, sitting supported.
2. Above plus sitting up in bed without support.
3. Above plus movements sitting over the edge of the bed and then in a chair.
4. Above plus walking around the room.
5. Above plus walking in the corridor and climbing a flight of stairs.
6. Above but dressed, plus walking out of doors.

At this point, the patient is fit to leave hospital. The time taken to get to stage 6 varies with each person – problems such as shortness of breath, chest pain, feeling faint, will delay progress to the next stage – and it can take anything from 10 days to 3 weeks. When leaving hospital the patient will benefit from some guidance, probably in the form of a booklet, on what he can do, for the 'limbo' period which occurs after discharge can be lonely and frightening. But having reached the stage of being able to climb stairs, the patient should be given positive advice, encouraging him to fit into the daily routine of home life as soon as possible.

Certainly he should read the papers and watch TV, but there is nothing to stop him from helping with the washing-up or flicking a duster about the place from very early on. It is a good idea to get outside, weather permitting – really cold weather and winds may cause chest pain – and walks should be planned according to the local geography. Walking is very important; it should be done two or three times a day, and it will relieve boredom and give the patient something positive to do. A suitable route should be mapped out, not too ambitious to start with – and not forgetting the return journey. Two hundred yards may be attempted very soon after getting home, and then if there are no problems increased slightly each day; the walk should not be taken too soon after a meal, and any problems such as chest pain or shortness of breath should be noted and reported to the doctor. A few weeks after the heart attack, up to half a mile taken at a fair pace, without getting too puffed or uncomfortable, would be very reasonable progress. Once this stage is reached the daily distance can be increased rapidly and activities generally broadened to include swinging a golf club, playing with the car, pottering in the garden in a more active way (greenhouse tending and light weeding can be done soon after discharge) so that, by the sixth week after the heart attack, life should be filling up and the scar left on the heart will have strengthened. If a formal rehabilitation programme is available, this is the time to start.

## Driving

There are two problems which are often raised at this time. The first is whether it is safe to drive a car. Driving is a potentially hazardous and stressful activity for the heart; considerable changes in pulse rate and blood pressure have been recorded in even an apparently uneventful journey. Simple procedures like negotiating roundabouts, road junctions and traffic jams can raise the pulse rate to levels equivalent to heavy exercise. So driving should be left until at least four weeks after the attack, and on the first few occasions it is worth taking a reliable companion who will boost confidence and be on hand should there be a mechanical failure or even a puncture, for changing a wheel or similar heavy procedure is not a good idea at this time. It is advisable also to avoid heavy traffic and all the frustrations that it entails.

## Sexual activity

The other frequent cause of worry is sexual potential, a problem still too often avoided in the general advice given after a heart attack. Often after a coronary the general feelings of loss of confidence, fear of death and inadequacy in the face of everyday living will show as an inability to perform sexually. As people are naturally reluctant to admit this, the problem is often not discussed; the general advice so often tossed out, 'Take it easy', may be interpreted as, 'Don't do it'.

One study of heart patients showed that two-thirds of them had a marked and lasting reduction in the frequency of intercourse. The reason for this in most cases was that none of them had had advice on what, if any, limitations should be put on their sex-life, and ignorance and fear in both partners plus a natural reluctance to admit or discuss any sexual inadequacy created an atmosphere of doubt in which it seemed easier and safer to restrict sexual activity – not a situation guaranteed to foster a happy relationship. Since most sexual activity involves two people, the partner should always be involved in any counselling, and fears, frustrations, tensions and difficulties may then be brought out into the open and discussed.

There is really no excuse for avoiding the subject now, as a great deal of work has been done on it. Admittedly much of the investigation took place under 'laboratory conditions' – hardly the most natural surroundings, with electrodes and wires on all parts of the anatomy – but with the more sophisticated electronic recording devices now available, the response of the heart during sexual activity has been accurately investigated.

The early papers on this subject produced evidence suggesting that the heart rate rose to 150 beats a minute. One investigation involved four leads made from wire mesh secured with elastic bandages to the upper thighs and upper arms, and to measure the breathing the subjects wore mouthpieces with valves; to make the results more accurate nose clamps were also worn and, as if this were not enough, buttons had to be pressed as intercourse progressed. It must also be remembered that most of these early investigations were done with young couples who had recently married or weren't married, some of whom had marital or sexual problems or were in other ways untypical.

More recent results were recorded from patients who had suffered a heart attack and were on the continuous twenty-four hour tape recorder mentioned earlier. In these patients, the average heart rate at orgasm was about 112, and about 85 beats per minute at 2 minutes before and 2 minutes after orgasm; when the heart-rate levels of this group were compared with their levels at work, the rates were much higher – averaging 120 beats per minute at maximum. An often quoted example is that of the lawyer whose heart rate during sexual activity was exceeded by his heart rate during his brisk walk to court, during his performance at the trial, when talking on the telephone with another lawyer and at dinner with his family.

Is there any evidence to show that the awful prospect, a deeply ingrained fear in many people's minds, of 'dying on the job' is a great deal less common than is generally assumed? The largest study done on this was in Japan; it showed that only 6 in 1000 episodes of sudden death were actually precipitated by sexual activity, and of these 77 per cent occurred during extra-marital episodes. So the possibility of dying from a coronary during intercourse with one's spouse seems very remote; extra-marital sex is clearly a different matter.

Intercourse is – besides other considerations – a form of physical exercise, so the better the state of general physical fitness, the easier and more enjoyable the exercise. Research in this field found that those patients who had been actively rehabilitated with a physical exercise programme after a heart attack had had sexual intercourse more frequently and with more enjoyment than those who had not been rehabilitated, and fewer of them complained of symptoms related to the heart – such as pain or heart flutter – during intercourse. The other partner can be of immeasurable help in this part of cardiac rehabilitation: a warm response made with confidence will do much to restore sexual identity and a sense of worth.

It is important not to over-indulge in food or alcohol before going to bed – this isn't a good idea anyway, and will add an additional load if intercourse follows too soon. As I have already implied, familiar surroundings and a familiar partner are a wise precaution in the early stages of rehabilitation. It is an integral part of the rehabilitation courses I have run to ask a man to bring his partner for a visit, for two reasons: first so that she can see the amount of physical work expected of him – this will reassure her that he is capable of leading a physically full life – and secondly, to discuss any problems she may have encountered as a result of his heart attack. Very often advice on sexual aspects is most welcome at this time.

As regards recommended positions of intercourse, it was suggested in the earlier studies that the male in the lower position or side to side would be least demanding; the male on top resembled the isometric type of exercise and was consequently more stressful. Recent studies using twenty-four hour tape-recorders at home have shown that difference in heart rate between the male being on top or underneath is virtually nil and that the blood pressure response was much the same, so it was concluded that position is not important as an added stress factor.

When to resume intercourse will of course vary with the individual, depending very much on the sexual appetite before the heart attack. As a general guideline, for the uncomplicated coronary with no symptoms after the acute stage, when two flights of stairs can be negotiated easily it is quite safe to have intercourse in marriage.

Intercourse, like any form of exercise, may bring on an attack of angina. Angina sufferers are advised to take a pain-relieving tablet – glyceryl tri-nitrate is usually prescribed – before any exercise they know will bring on the pain. These should always be close at hand, and the side of the bed is no exception; they should be easily accessible – not hidden in a box in a drawer, necessitating much groping at the critical moment, but easily at hand. Angina is *not* a sign of impending doom, but a symptom of oxygen deficiency which can be quickly relieved, and is no reason for ceasing activity and leaving two unfulfilled, frustrated people.

Although most of my comments have referred to male sexual problems, many of them obviously apply to women who have suffered heart attacks: sexual drive, changes in the pattern of intercourse and the heart output, and fears associated with these are the same for both sexes. Both partners must be understanding and patient, allowing each other time to adjust and accept the situation. In the long term, such patience and understanding will be rewarded by a relationship unimpaired by the sexual difficulties so often associated with heart attacks.

# Physical training programme

About six weeks after a heart attack a follow-up visit to the hospital is usually arranged, at which the physician will review the patient's general condition and progress. Unfortunately in Britain, due to lack of finance, many hospitals are unable to offer more than general advice for the future at this visit; in this case physical progress must be undertaken along the lines I have mentioned earlier, with a booklet of advice and some idea of the milestones to be aimed for, under the guidance and encouragement of the family doctor. Sometimes the hospital physician may recommend a formal course of rehabilitation aimed at improving the physical fitness and confidence of the patient; this may take one of several forms depending on the staff and funds available. The exercise prescription will vary from centre to centre, but every case must be assessed on its own merits; the patient who has had an uncomplicated attack with no symptoms after it can usually – but not always – be treated more vigorously than someone suffering from angina, shortness of breath, and so on.

The programme may be run in individual sessions (not usually very practical), in groups of 2 or 3 people, or in classes of up to 20, depending on the time and facilities available. Attendance should be at least two or three times a week, and most would agree three times to be the ideal; if once a week only is possible, advice must be given after each session as to what activity should be undertaken before the next session. Ideally, for the first few sessions anyway, the patient is kept on monitor control, and the most convenient way to do this is by using a radio-telemetry unit (described on page 82). In this case the patient wears a belt containing a small box – the transmitter – to which are attached leads from three electrodes attached to the chest; these transmit the electrical activity of the heart to the receiver which converts the signal to an ECG on the television monitor. In this way the patient is mobile, and the heart rate and rhythm can be constantly observed while he is undertaking a variety of physical activities. Unfortunately this is a very expensive piece of electrical wizardry and its priority on the NHS budget is very low. If monitoring is not available by telemetry it is advisable that an exercise test (see page 81) be performed before a programme of physical training is recommended; this will give the physician enough information on which to base his exercise prescription. Even if neither monitoring nor exercise testing is possible, a great deal of benefit can be obtained from a programme in which the pulse rates only are measured. In this case it is advisable not to allow the pulse rate to exceed 120 to start with, and less in the elderly or those receiving medication such as beta blockers.

## Isometric and isotonic exercise

Isometric exercise is that in which the muscle fibres remain at the same length; it involves static contraction and no joint movement – for example, bracing a muscle or pushing against a closed door. These muscle-building exercises have very little benefit on the heart muscle, and indeed prolonged contraction of the muscles can cause a fall in supply of blood to the heart and raise the blood pressure. However, since day-to-day living inevitably involves some isometric movements – lifting luggage, carrying trays, pushing doors – it is important that the patient should be able to cope with these demands.

In isotonics, or dynamic exercise – running or cycling, for example – the muscle fibres lengthen and shorten. This increases the heart rate and output and is the basis on which exercise rehabilitation is built; it is not a programme to make a 'body beautiful' with bulging muscles, nor to reduce weight and produce a new svelte you, but a programme devised and prescribed to improve the efficiency of the heart.

Any form of repetitive physical exercise can be boring and for this reason the programme has a variety of exercises, all designed to increase the heart rate and efficiency. The exercising equipment, as with the monitoring facilities, will largely depend on the budget, but the success of the course depends not so much on the equipment available as on the enthusiasm of the individual running the course, whether this be a doctor, physiotherapist or nurse. Without such enthusiasm patients will become discouraged and drop out: the drop-out rate, which varies from 1 to 30 per cent, depends very much on the atmosphere of the individual unit.

Time should be given during the first visits to explain just what the aims of the course are. There is a widespread and deep-seated misconception that 'heart attacks should rest', and the sight of exercise bicycles, treadmills and rowing machines is often viewed with suspicion and apprehension. A few minutes' explanation of each piece of equipment, why it is there and what its function is, will clear many of these feelings of fear. If this is done on an individual basis, queries will not be inhibited and the point of the treatment will be understood; questions should be encouraged, and then answered truthfully and knowledgeably so that individual trust and confidence is developed.

It is impossible to cover here all the various types of rehabilitation course available, but it may be helpful to describe some of the equipment which will be present.

*Cycle ergometer* – a static bike. Most people will have seen one of these at some time or another: basically it consists of pedals linked to a wheel which can be made to work against friction, either by a brake pad or by a friction belt. There is an enormous variety of design, and the cost is related to the sophistication and calibration of the mechanics of the bike; the most expensive are highly accurate pieces of scientific equipment on which a great deal of investigation into the effect of exercise on the heart has been made, particularly in Scandinavia. The friction is usually adjustable, and often a work table is provided which gives an indication of how much physical effort is needed at a predetermined loading. A small amount of skill is needed to use the cycle ergometer: it will be no problem to anyone who has cycled before, but for someone who has never ridden a bicycle – and surprisingly there are some who have never even sat on one – the rhythm required to turn the pedals sometimes proves difficult to learn.

*Rowing machine.* This consists of a seat on runners or a rail, a footplate, often with a strap to help keep the feet steady, and two handles attached to springs or plungers. The movement is similar to that of rowing a boat, and involves sitting forward then pulling back on the handles and straightening the legs. There is an isometric element about this exercise, which is useful in preparation for isometric movements involved in ordinary living.

*Step*. Stepping exercises have been used for years in investigating the heart's response to exercise. What is known as the 'two-step' procedure was first used before the war, and has proved its value ever since. The height of the step varies – in physiotherapy departments, the low is about 23cm (9 inches) high – and the movement involves putting one foot up on the stool or step and then the other, lowering one foot and then the other; to keep the timing constant, this can be done to a metronome setting or even to music.

A very useful, newer version of the step is adjustable: the step takes the form of a tray which slides into a box, with runners at varying heights. The setting should be such that, with the flat of the foot on the step, the thigh is parallel to the ground; in this way the step can be adjusted to the individual's height and the work-load may later be increased by the level at which the tray or step is placed. Wall bars above the box may be used to help keep the balance.

*Weights*. These should be used with caution as the exercise involved is totally isometric. The weights should not be so heavy as to cause straining when lifted, as this lowers the efficiency of the heart and increases blood pressure. There are several types of weight: individually hand held or barbells, or those pulled against a weight on a wall. All of them should be approached with the same caution, but they can be useful, particularly when preparing someone for return to certain light manual jobs such as painting and decorating.

*Treadmill.* The treadmill is a very expensive but highly accurate and useful part of the equipment for both exercise testing and rehabilitation. Most exercise testing is now performed on this machine, which can usually be varied in gradient and speed. In the rehabilitation programme it can be used as part of the exercise circuit; it can be adjusted to suit each individual case and can be made as easy or difficult as necessary.

There are two major problems with the treadmill: first the expense – particularly in Britain few rehabilitation units have one – and secondly that it requires a certain co-ordination and skill which some people find difficult to achieve.

So much for the exercising equipment which may be used to increase heart rate and output; in order to estimate this, recording and monitoring equipment may include the following.

*Pulse monitor.* There are a number of gadgets on the market which will record the pulse rate electronically: one works by a finger being inserted into a clip with a photo-electric cell; another more robust machine has handles which are gripped and the pulse rate is recorded on a dial. They are not essential pieces of equipment but are useful for classes, when several readings will need to be taken for each person attending.

It is useful for people on these courses to learn to take their own pulse, not only to streamline the course itself, but so that during their own home programme they can assess their own performance. The only equipment needed is a watch with a second hand. The pulse is taken by placing the index and middle fingertips on the outer, lower aspect of the opposite forearm, just above the wrist, with the hand facing upwards; right-handed people usually wear a watch on the left arm, so will use the left fingers on the right forearm – left-handed people the other way round. With light pressure, the pulse can be felt beneath the fingers and counted while the second hand on the watch moves round for 15 seconds. The count multiplied by four gives the number of beats per minute and is an acceptably accurate pulse measurement.

*Monitoring equipment.* There are many types of monitoring equipment for watching cardiac activity. They vary in size and the amount of information they provide, but they all have a screen called an oscilloscope: this is similar to a television screen and shows the heart's activity and re-action to stress. The activity of the heart is represented as a line on the screen, with a typical pattern which changes on exercise. These changes themselves have a characteristic pattern, both in normal activity and in abnormal rhythm due to overloading of the heart. For this reason it is useful to monitor patients early in a rehabilitation course, so that the effects of exercise can be closely watched and the exercise prescription changed if necessary.

The signal can be transmitted from the heart to the monitor either by radio-telemetry or by a direct link with wires attached from the chest to the monitor; radio-telemetry, already described on page 82, is of course pre-ferable as it allows much greater freedom of movement. These machines have been used in studying hearts at very high levels of exercise and stress, such as during ski-jumping and motor-racing. The advantage of the direct link monitor is that although it will restrict the amount of movement made by the subject, it will in many cases produce a better write-out in which any variations of the pattern may be easier to detect.

The oscilloscope itself will not give a permanent record of any changes that may occur, so it is linked to a writer – a heated stylus which reproduces the line on the oscilloscope on a heat-sensitive paper which is running at a speed previously set and standardized. This enables a permanent record to be kept which can be studied and compared with previous records; in this way it is possible to compare heart function over a period of time and to follow progress.

*Resuscitation equipment.* Tucked away in one corner of the exercise room, but easily accessible, will be the resuscitation equipment – known in the United States as a 'crash-cart'. This is *not* to be looked upon as something which will be used frequently – it most certainly will not be – but as a source of reassurance that everything is on hand to deal with an emergency. The most noticeable object is the defibrillator (see page 65) – probably red and looking like a small fire extinguisher; there will also be an oxygen cylinder and mask and a tray of syringes and ampoules.

So, having familiarized himself with the aims of the course, its situation and equipment, the patient can start some work. What this entails will vary with the facilities available and the preferences of the person running the course.

## Monitored exercises

There are only a few units in Britain where exercise is monitored by oscilloscope, largely because of lack of funds; the great advantage of this method is that whoever is running the course can see exactly what is happening to the heart as it happens.

The transmitter or direct lines are fixed to the chest with small electrodes on an adhesive plastic cuff, and once a satisfactory signal appears on the monitor, the exercise can start. A warming-up period is usually a good idea, and this can be done on the cycle ergometer, just moving the pedals round with no friction applied to start with then applying a low friction for a very short time at a steady rate of pedalling; most ergometers have a speedometer and the predetermined rate must be maintained. Some muscle fatigue is inevitable, but any other untoward symptoms such as shortness of breath or chest pain should be declared – not 'bravely borne' – and the exercise stopped if necessary. Usually the work-loads given at the beginning are so low that they present no problems. At the end of the set time – usually as short as $1\frac{1}{2}$ minutes to start with – the pulse rate is read off from the monitor, on either a write-out or digital display, and recorded.

Provided the pulse is within acceptable limits the exercise will be repeated after a short rest, and if the first session was found to be too easy the resistance of the cycle may be increased. This early session is important in order to establish a baseline of exercise which is satisfactory to both doctor and patient: too easy and there will be no benefit, too difficult and the patient will feel that he won't be able to cope with the course.

What is an acceptable pulse rate? Much of the progress of the course depends on pulse response, and this varies with each individual – indeed each individual will have varying responses, particularly of the resting pulse, to emotion, frustration, smoking and so on. Tables have been produced giving the predicted heart rates of a normal population (see page 126); the maximum rate possible to attain falls with age, and some programmes will use these tables to set a target of the predicted maximum for age. Such programmes tend to be rather extreme, and a more generally accepted target would be 120–130 beats per minute. Even this will sometimes not be possible, as many of the drugs used after heart attacks prevent the heart from beating at more than 120 beats per minute however much exercise is required.

## Averages of maximum heart rates

| Age | 25 | 30 | 35 | 40 | 45 | 50 | 55 | 60 | 65 |
|---|---|---|---|---|---|---|---|---|---|
| Maximum heart rate (MHR) | 190 | 186 | 182 | 181 | 179 | 175 | 171 | 168 | 164 |
| 90% MHR | 171 | 167 | 164 | 163 | 161 | 158 | 154 | 151 | 148 |
| 85% MHR | 162 | 158 | 155 | 154 | 152 | 149 | 145 | 143 | 139 |
| 80% MHR | 152 | 149 | 146 | 145 | 143 | 140 | 137 | 134 | 131 |
| 75% MHR | 143 | 140 | 137 | 136 | 134 | 131 | 128 | 126 | 123 |
| 70% MHR | 133 | 130 | 127 | 127 | 125 | 123 | 120 | 118 | 115 |
| 65% MHR | 124 | 121 | 118 | 118 | 116 | 114 | 111 | 109 | 107 |
| 60% MHR | 114 | 112 | 109 | 109 | 107 | 105 | 103 | 101 | 98 |

Once the preliminary session is over, the patient can be introduced to the circuit; this will prevent boredom and introduce alternative ways of exercising. A typical circuit would be to start on the cycle, then use the rowing machine, the treadmill, the step and finish perhaps with another trip on the cycle. Each exercise period will work up to 3 minutes, giving a total of 15 minutes' exercise; this will be mainly dynamic isotonic, but with an element of isometrics in the rowing machine to provide some preparation for everyday living.

Careful records must be kept of the work-load and pulse rate after each exercise so that the course can be adapted according to individual responses; these will show that, as body fitness – part of which is heart fitness – improves, the pulse rate for a given amount of work will gradually decrease, showing that the heart is becoming a more efficient pump. As the course progresses, work-loads will be steadily increased and physical capabilities improved, and with this improvement will come a marked feeling of general wellbeing and confidence.

No athlete in training expects to reach his goal quickly – he knows that a long, slow build-up is the best way to reach his target. So it is with training a heart: it is quite useless to have a vigorous bout of exercise and then do nothing about it for the rest of the week, and ideally exercise sessions in a course of treatment should be provided on 3 days a week, giving a total of 45 minutes of exercise weekly for at least 6 and preferably 10 weeks.

One of the possible disadvantages of a monitored programme is that a patient may become dependent on the monitor for his confidence, feeling that only as long as someone is watching his heart in action, can nothing go wrong. For this reason, once the work-loads are increasing and providing there is no medical reason for retaining it, the oscilloscope can be dispensed with, and the monitoring done by pulse rates only.

Many of the benefits of a cardiac rehabilitation course of exercise are subjective, and it is very difficult to measure how well a person feels. But the results of all courses show clearly an improvement in morale and confidence (possibly because the responsibility for getting better is partially transferred to someone else's shoulders), and positive advice on what can be done and how to do it is far more acceptable and constructive than the so often given, negative advice of 'Take it easy and see how it goes'. The road of trial and error is a frightening one, and most people will vere to the more conservative side which makes progress slow and laborious and does little to enhance sagging confidence. At the end of the course the patient should have an accurate awareness of his capabilities, and limitations – if any are needed – must be outlined with care and accuracy.

The physical improvement can be charted by repeat exercise testing (the methods for this are described on page 83): the first test is performed early on in the course, after the patient is familiar with and settled into the programme, and the heart rates achieved are plotted on a graph against the work-load required to reach this rate; the second test is performed at the end of the course using exactly the same times and work-loads, and the results are plotted on the same chart. From this chart it is easy to see that to produce the previous pulse levels, quite a lot more work has to be undertaken in the second test – clearly the heart has become a much more efficient machine. This is a very satisfying moment for both patient and doctor, and a justification for all the previous weeks of effort.

## Non-monitored rehabilitation courses

The disadvantage of the monitored course is the expense in terms of equipment and personnel, as relatively few people can be dealt with at any one time. But excellent results can be obtained without sophisticated equipment and with a criterion of quality rather than quantity for personnel. Whether the person running the course is a doctor, physiotherapist, remedial gymnast, trained nurse or occupational therapist, he or she must have enthusiasm and confidence and be able to transmit these qualities to those taking part. Whoever is in charge there should always be either a doctor on call or a team who can deal with any emergency, and in any case it is a good idea for a doctor to visit fairly frequently, so that he can answer queries on medical problems from the patients or their relatives.

A non-monitored course may be run as a class and thus provide 'self-help' to a greater number of people. Exercises can be performed on stools, benches, wall-bars, with dumb-bells, or even just jogging; each patient will take and record his own pulse either by hand as described or by a special pulse recording machine (see page 122). The target heart rate will be set by the person running the course and, as in the monitored course, any untoward symptoms must be reported at once.

The amount of exercise performed will vary with the kind of course and with the attitude of the person running it – one trial in which a comparable group was split into three sections showed that the general improvement in confidence and wellbeing was the same overall, whether the course had involved strenuous or mild exercise.

## Home programme

The end of the course is really the beginning of the rehabilitation for the patient. By then he will have reached a level of general physical fitness which will give him a good quality of life, but – just as for an athlete – stop the training and the fitness will diminish rapidly. So keeping up the training should become as much of a habit as cleaning your teeth. Exercise may be done outside or inside, although outside gives more opportunity for such excuses as 'I'll skip it today or else I'll get double pneumonia in this weather', and, as already stated, particularly cold weather or winds may bring on angina.

The simplest and cheapest way of exercising indoors is using a step; a reasonable height is 45cm (18 inches) and the form of exercise is simply to step on and off as described on page 121; 20 to 24 cycles should be done in one minute and the exercise continued for 3 minutes.

Some people will prefer to buy a rowing machine or static bike, or to jog; it doesn't really matter which sort of exercise is chosen as long as the general rules in relation to timing, regularity and pulse rates are followed.

# Some practical guidance

The following are guidelines on a home programme of rehabilitation given by The Council on Rehabilitation of The International Society of Cardiology in 1973. They provide sensible and straightforward advice on which to build your own programme.

1. If you are at work, the best available times for exercise are before work in the morning, after returning from work and before the evening meal, or some time after the meal before going to bed.

2. A considerable walk to work may fill the requirements of daily exercise; if your work is a heavy manual job, this in itself may be enough regular exercise.

3. The aim is to maintain reasonable physical fitness rather than to achieve an athletic standard.

4. Sudden or prolonged unaccustomed exercise is harmful and could even be dangerous.

5. A specific, regular route and distance followed from time to time is useful as a 'pacer', to compare performance and assess improvement or possibly deterioration.

6. Don't exercise for at least 2 hours after a main meal.

7. Don't exercise if you are unwell or overtired – take time to get over a cold before restarting regular exercises.

8. On holiday, continue regular training but substitute swimming or other exercises for normal exercise if you like.

9. In building up the work-load, increase first the duration then the pace, and do both gradually.

10. Let someone else do the really heavy work – especially if this involves isometrics such as pushing a car, carrying a heavy stone, heavy spadework and so on.

11. If angina, undue breathlessness, palpitations or other untoward symptoms occur during exercise, reduce speed;

if this is not effective, stop and rest. If angina does occur, get into the habit of carrying nitro-glycerine tablets.

12. After exercise you should have a satisfying feeling of wellbeing. If this doesn't happen you have probably exceeded the correct level of speed or duration, or perhaps you have exercised in unsuitable weather. Whatever the reason, you should adjust to an acceptable level of exercise.

13. If you take a bath or shower after exercise, make sure the water is comfortably warm – neither too hot nor too cold.

14. If you experience any giddiness, lightheadedness, unpleasant palpitations, 'leaden legs', or new chest discomfort you should report this to the doctor (remembering that if you stand still immediately after exercise some of these symptoms will naturally appear).

15. Unpleasant pain in the joints or muscles is usually the result of excessive exertion. Reduce the intensity of the exercise until the affected muscles are 'trained'.

16. It is advisable to have a medical check-up once or twice a year.

# Conclusion: Some Facts and Figures

In Britain attempts at public education on coronary artery disease are failing – whether this is because of a general apathy or real disbelief in the facts is difficult to say. It is hoped that this book will help to clarify much of the mystique associated with the disease and the investigations involved in accurate diagnosis.

There has been a primary prevention programme of education to reduce coronary disease in the United States for some years. The British may view this with a certain amount of scepticism, but the facts speak for themselves. The programme teaches the significance of risk factors, and probably the best known result of this is what could be called a new cult – jogging. Well, cult or not, the facts are undeniable. The following figures were quoted at the American Heart Association Convention in Miami Beach in 1977:

For the first time since 1964 there were less than 1,000,000 heart attacks in the United States.

In 1975 (the latest figure available) there were 38,000 fewer people dying from heart attacks than in 1970.

Since 1956 the rate per 100,000 adult males dropped by 30 per cent.

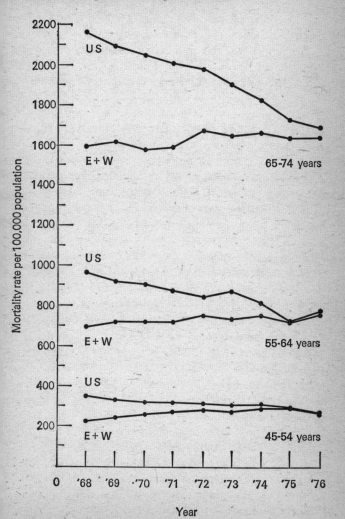

**Mortality trends from coronary heart disease in men in the US and England + Wales 1968-1976**

Mortality rate per 100,000 population

US

E + W

65-74 years

US

E + W

55-64 years

US

E + W

45-54 years

0   '68   '69   '70   '71   '72   '73   '74   '75   '76

Year

In Britain, the figures from the Registrar General show that nearly 1000 people a day die from diseases of the heart and circulatory disorders. This is two and a half times more than the number dying from all forms of cancer and twice the number of deaths from all other causes.

The trend is clear: sufferers from coronary artery disease are not members of an élite club, but of one which is grossly over-subscribed and with numbers rising rapidly. A good education programme, diligently followed, can definitely help to reduce the membership.

Most people are lazy by nature and all too prepared to look for and find reasons why a small change in lifestyle is not possible for them. Excuses range from 'I haven't the time', when talking about exercise, to the favourite excuse for not doing anything about obesity: 'What can I do? My business involves such a lot of entertaining.'

People need convincing that 30 minutes of dynamic exercise a week is sufficient to keep the heart in good condition (is there anyone who cannot spare 10 minutes three times a week?) and a glance at the calorie charts on page 140 will show that most menus have a vast range of low calorie foods for those who want them.

Stress, the third main risk factor, comes in a variety of guises – business deadlines, financial worries and so on. Some stress is of course unavoidable, indeed a certain amount is healthy, but a great deal is self-generated. None of us is as indispensable as we like to think: life will go on without us, and it is well worth while sitting back and taking stock of how well or badly your life is organized – then taking positive steps to improve things.

Some risk factors are not clearly apparent to the individual and may need expert investigation. The most important of these is raised blood pressure, which is commonly only found at medical examination; it takes a doctor very little time to discover this potent risk factor which can often be controlled with medication. Much the same applies to lipids and cholesterol blood levels: it is a relatively minor matter to have some blood taken and examined, and if the levels are raised to deal with the problem either by diet alone or diet with some medication.

The formation of atheromatous plaques is not a rapid process, but one which will progress relentlessly if we ignore the factors which encourage it. Damage already there will not regress, but progression can be slowed down if we will only take the trouble to kick the bad habits that most of us acquire in adult life.

## Desirable weights

### Men

| Height | | Small frame | | Medium frame | | Large frame | |
|---|---|---|---|---|---|---|---|
| ft | in | lb | kg | lb | kg | lb | kg |
| 5 | 1 | 112–120 | 51–55 | 118–129 | 54–59 | 126–141 | 57–64 |
| 5 | 2 | 115–123 | 52–56 | 121–133 | 55–60 | 129–144 | 59–65 |
| 5 | 3 | 118–126 | 54–57 | 124–136 | 56–62 | 132–148 | 60–67 |
| 5 | 4 | 121–124 | 55–59 | 127–131 | 58–63 | 135–152 | 61–69 |
| 5 | 5 | 124–133 | 56–60 | 130–143 | 59–65 | 138–156 | 63–71 |
| 5 | 6 | 128–137 | 58–62 | 134–147 | 61–67 | 142–161 | 65–73 |
| 5 | 7 | 132–141 | 60–64 | 138–152 | 63–69 | 147–166 | 67–75 |
| 5 | 8 | 136–145 | 62–66 | 142–156 | 65–71 | 151–170 | 69–77 |
| 5 | 9 | 140–150 | 64–68 | 146–160 | 66–73 | 155–174 | 70–79 |
| 5 | 10 | 144–154 | 65–70 | 150–165 | 68–75 | 159–179 | 72–81 |
| 5 | 11 | 148–158 | 67–72 | 154–170 | 70–77 | 164–184 | 75–84 |
| 6 | 0 | 152–162 | 69–74 | 158–175 | 72–80 | 168–189 | 76–86 |
| 6 | 1 | 156–167 | 71–76 | 162–180 | 74–82 | 173–194 | 79–88 |
| 6 | 2 | 160–171 | 73–78 | 167–185 | 76–84 | 178–199 | 81–90 |
| 6 | 3 | 164–175 | 75–80 | 172–190 | 78–86 | 182–204 | 83–93 |

### Women

| Height | | Small frame | | Medium frame | | Large frame | |
|---|---|---|---|---|---|---|---|
| ft | in | lb | kg | lb | kg | lb | kg |
| 4 | 8 | 92–98 | 42–45 | 96–107 | 44–49 | 104–119 | 47–54 |
| 4 | 9 | 94–101 | 43–46 | 98–110 | 45–50 | 106–122 | 48–55 |
| 4 | 10 | 96–104 | 44–47 | 101–113 | 46–51 | 109–125 | 50–57 |
| 4 | 11 | 99–107 | 45–49 | 104–116 | 47–53 | 112–128 | 51–58 |
| 5 | 0 | 102–110 | 46–50 | 107–119 | 49–54 | 115–131 | 52–60 |
| 5 | 1 | 105–113 | 48–51 | 110–122 | 50–55 | 118–134 | 54–61 |
| 5 | 2 | 108–116 | 49–53 | 113–126 | 51–57 | 121–138 | 55–63 |
| 5 | 3 | 111–119 | 51–54 | 116–130 | 53–59 | 125–142 | 57–65 |
| 5 | 4 | 114–123 | 52–56 | 120–135 | 55–61 | 129–146 | 59–66 |
| 5 | 5 | 118–127 | 54–58 | 124–139 | 56–63 | 133–150 | 60–68 |
| 5 | 6 | 122–131 | 55–60 | 128–143 | 58–65 | 137–154 | 62–70 |
| 5 | 7 | 126–135 | 57–61 | 132–147 | 60–67 | 141–158 | 64–72 |
| 5 | 8 | 130–140 | 59–64 | 136–151 | 62–69 | 145–163 | 66–74 |
| 5 | 9 | 134–144 | 61–65 | 140–155 | 64–70 | 149–168 | 68–76 |
| 5 | 10 | 138–148 | 63–67 | 144–159 | 65–72 | 153–173 | 70–79 |

*Note: These weights include indoor clothing, i.e. 5–7 lb for men's clothes, 2–4 lb for women's.*

# Unit eating guide

*This method of dieting depends on reducing to a minimum the amount of carbohydrate eaten. You may eat what you like of foods in Group 1, and aim for a maximum of 12 units a day from Groups 2 and 3*

## Group 1
*No units – eat as much as you like*

**Vegetables**
Beans, green
Broccoli
Brussels sprouts
Cabbage
Cauliflower
Celery
Cucumber
Leeks
Lettuce
Mushrooms
Onions
Spinach
Tomatoes
Watercress

**Fats and oils**
Lard
Suet
Mayonnaise
Oil, cooking
  salad

**Dairy products**
Butter
Margarine
Cheese (all sorts)
Cream

**Meat**
Bacon
Beef
Chicken
Duck
Game
Ham
Heart
Kidneys
Lamb, mutton
Liver
Pork
Tongue
Tripe
Turkey
Veal

**Fish and shellfish**
Bloaters
Crab
Eel
Flatfish
Herrings
Kippers
Lobster
Mackerel
Mussels
Oysters
Pilchards
Prawns
Roe
Salmon
Sardines
Sprats
Trout
Tuna

**Beverages**
All 'low calorie' drinks
Coffee (black)
Tea (black)

## Group 2
*Caution – eat in moderation*

| Fruit | Average portion | Units |
|---|---|---|
| Apples | one | 2 |
| Apricots, fresh | 4 oz | 1 |
| Cherries | 4 oz | 3 |
| Figs, fresh | 4 oz | 3 |
| Gooseberries | 4 oz | 2 |
| Grapefruit | half | 1 |
| Melon | 6 oz | 2 |
| Oranges | 6 oz | 3 |
| Peaches, fresh | 4 oz | 1 |
| Pears, fresh | 5 oz | $2\frac{1}{2}$ |
| Pineapple, fresh | 4 oz | 2 |
| Plums, fresh | 4 oz | 2 |
| Raisins | 1 oz | 3 |
| Raspberries | 4 oz | 2 |

| Vegetables | Average portion | Units |
|---|---|---|
| Avocado pear | half | 1 |
| Beans, baked | 4 oz | 4 |
| broad | 4 oz | 3 |
| butter | 4 oz | 4 |
| haricot | 4 oz | 4 |
| kidney | 1 oz | 4 |
| Beetroot | 2 oz | 1 |
| Carrots | 3 oz | 1 |
| Parsnips | 4 oz | 2 |
| Peas | 4 oz | 2 |
| Swede | 4 oz | 1 |
| Turnips | 3 oz | 1 |

| Nuts | Average portion | Units |
|---|---|---|
| Brazil | 10 | $\frac{1}{2}$ |
| Cashew | 1 oz | $1\frac{1}{2}$ |
| Coconut | 2 oz | 3 |
| Hazel | 15 | $\frac{1}{2}$ |
| Peanuts | 30 | 1 |
| Walnuts | 10 | $\frac{1}{2}$ |

| Cereals and cereal products | Average portion | Units |
|---|---|---|
| Bread, starch reduced | 1 oz | 2 |
| Energen, roll | 1 oz | $\frac{1}{2}$ |
| crispbread | 1 piece | $\frac{1}{2}$ |
| Flour, soya | 1 oz | 1 |

| Fats and oils | Average portion | Units |
|---|---|---|
| Peanut butter | 1 oz | 1 |

| Dairy products | Average portion | Units |
|---|---|---|
| Milk, evaporated | 2 oz | 1 |
| fresh* | $\frac{1}{2}$ pint | 3 |
| Yoghurt, plain | 5 oz | 1 |

*Because milk is so rich in nutrients, at least $\frac{1}{2}$ pint should be drunk each day*

| Meat | Average portion | Units |
|---|---|---|
| Sausages, fresh | each | 2 |
| Stew | 4 oz | 2 |

| Beverages | Average portion | Units |
|---|---|---|
| Orange juice, unsweetened | 4 oz | 2 |
| Ovaltine | 1 tblsp | 1 |
| Pineapple juice | 4 oz | $2\frac{1}{2}$ |
| Tomato juice | 3 oz | 1 |

## Group 3
*Danger — avoid where possible*

| Fruit | Average portion | Units |
|---|---|---|
| Bananas | one | 5 |
| Dates, dried | 1 oz | 4 |
| Figs, dried | 1 oz | 3 |
| in syrup | 4 oz | 8 |
| Grapes | 4 oz | 3 |
| Mandarins, in syrup | 4 oz | 4 |
| Other tinned fruits in syrup | 4 oz | 5 |

| Vegetables | Average portion | Units |
|---|---|---|
| Corn-on-the-cob | 4 oz | 4 |
| Potato | 3 oz | 3 |
| crisps | 1 oz | 3 |
| Sweet potatoes | 3 oz | 5 |

| Cereals and cereal products | Average portion | Units |
|---|---|---|
| Biscuits, plain | 3 | 3 |
| sweet | 2 | 3 |
| Bread, brown, white | 1 oz | 3 |
| Breakfast cereals | 1 oz | 5 |
| Cake | 2 oz | 7 |
| Cornflour | 1 oz | 5 |
| Custard | 4 oz | 2 |
| Flour | 1 oz | 4 |
| Macaroni, boiled | 6 oz | 10 |
| Milk pudding | 4 oz | 5 |
| Papadum | one | 7 |
| Pastry | 1 oz | 3 |
| Rice, cooked | 4 oz | 5 |
| Vermicelli, cooked | 6 oz | 9 |
| Yorkshire pudding | 2 oz | 5 |

| Puddings and pies | Average portion | Units |
|---|---|---|
| Apple dumplings | 4 oz | 4 |

| | Average portion | Units |
|---|---|---|
| Apple pie | 4 oz | 7 |
| Ice cream | 2 oz | 3 |
| Jelly | 4 oz | 4 |
| Mince pies | 2 oz | 5 |
| Pancakes | 2 oz | 4 |
| Plum pudding | 3 oz | 9 |
| Rhubarb pie | 4 oz | 6 |

| Beverages | Average portion | Units |
|---|---|---|
| Ale, beer, lager | ½ pint | 5 |
| Brandy | 1 oz | 4 |
| Cider | ½ pint | 7 |
| Gin | 1 oz | 4 |
| Lemonade | 8 oz | 5 |
| Liqueurs | 1 oz | 5 |
| Lucozade | 6 oz | 6 |
| Orange juice, sweetened | 4 oz | 3 |
| Sherry | 2 oz | 4 |
| Tonic water | 6 oz | 2½ |
| Vermouth, dry | 2 oz | 3 |
| sweet | 2 oz | 5 |
| Whisky | 1 oz | 4 |
| Wine, dry | 3 oz | 3 |
| sweet | 3 oz | 4 |

| Sweets, etc. | Average portion | Units |
|---|---|---|
| Chocolate | 2 oz | 5 |
| Golden syrup | 1 oz | 4 |
| Honey | 1 oz | 5 |
| Jam | ½ oz | 2 |
| Sugar, brown, white | ½ oz | 3 |
| Sweets, boiled | 1 oz | 4 |

*Note: 1 oz = 30 grams approx.*

# Calories

| Fruit | Average portion | No. of calories |
|---|---|---|
| Apples | one | 60 |
| Apricots, fresh | 4 oz | 32 |
| in syrup | 4 oz | 120 |
| dried, raw | 2 oz | 104 |
| Bananas | 1 (4 oz) | 88 |
| Gooseberries | 4 oz | 40 |
| Grapefruit | ½ (4 oz) | 12 |
| Grapes | 3 oz | 51 |
| Melon | 6 oz | 24–42 |
| Oranges | 1 (6 oz) | 60 |
| Peaches, fresh | 1 (4 oz) | 44 |
| in syrup | 4 oz | 100 |
| Pears, fresh | 1 (5 oz) | 45 |
| in syrup | 4 oz | 88 |
| Pineapple, fresh | 4 oz | 52 |
| in syrup | 4 oz | 88 |
| Plums, fresh | 2 oz | 20 |
| in syrup | 4 oz | 88 |
| Raisins | 1 oz | 70 |
| Raspberries | 4 oz | 28 |
| Rhubarb | 4 oz | 8 |

| Vegetables | Average portion | No. of calories |
|---|---|---|
| Beans, baked | 4 oz | 104 |
| broad | 4 oz | 48 |
| French | 4 oz | 8 |
| haricot, boiled | 4 oz | 100 |
| Beetroot, boiled | 2 oz | 26 |
| Broccoli | 4 oz | 16 |
| Brussels sprouts | 3 oz | 15 |
| Cabbage, boiled | 4 oz | 8 |
| Carrots | 3 oz | 18 |
| Cauliflower | 4 oz | 12 |
| Celery, raw | 3 oz | 9 |
| Cucumber | 2 oz | 6 |
| Leeks | 4 oz | 28 |
| Lentils, dried | 1½ oz | 104 |
| Lettuce | ¼ oz | 1 |
| Mushrooms | 2 oz | 4 |
| Onions, boiled | 4 oz | 16 |
| fried | 2 oz | 202 |
| Parsnips | 4 oz | 64 |
| Peas | 4 oz | 56 |
| Potatoes, boiled | 4 oz | 92 |

| | Average portion | No. of calories |
|---|---|---|
| chips | 4 oz | 272 |
| crisps | 1 oz | 159 |
| roast | 4 oz | 140 |
| Spinach | 4 oz | 28 |
| Swede, boiled | 4 oz | 20 |
| Tomatoes | 4 oz | 16 |
| Turnips | 3 oz | 9 |

| Nuts | Average portion | No. of calories |
|---|---|---|
| Various, dried | 1 oz | 156–189 |
| Chestnuts, fresh | 2 oz | 96 |

| Cereals and cereal products | Average portion | No. of calories |
|---|---|---|
| Biscuits, plain | 2 oz | 226 |
| sweet | 2 oz | 316 |
| Bread | 1 slice | 65–72 |
| buttered | 1 slice | 135 |
| fried | 1 slice | 185 |
| Breakfast cereals | 1 oz | 100/104 |
| Cake, fruit | 2 oz | 220/282 |
| Cornflour | 1 oz | 100 |
| Custard | 4 oz | 128 |
| Energen rolls | 2 | 36 |
| Flour | 1 oz | 100 |
| Macaroni, boiled | 1 oz | 32 |
| Milk puddings | 8 oz | 320 |
| Oatmeal, raw | 1 oz | 115 |
| Pastry, shortcrust | 2 oz | 280 |
| Ryvita | 2 | 68 |
| Spaghetti, canned, in tomato sauce | 4 oz | 70 |
| Yorkshire pudding | 4 oz | 252 |

| Fats | Average portion | No. of calories |
|---|---|---|
| Lard and suet | ½ oz | 65 |
| Mayonnaise | ½ oz | 103 |
| Peanut butter | ¼ oz | 43 |

| Dairy products | Average portion | No. of calories |
|---|---|---|
| Cheese | | |
| Camembert, | | |
| Edam | 1½ oz | 132 |
| Cheddar | 1½ oz | 180 |
| cottage | 1½ oz | 45 |

| | Average portion | No. of calories | | Average portion | No. of calories |
|---|---|---|---|---|---|
| cream | 1½ oz | 348 | Pilchards, canned | 4 oz | 216 |
| Gorgonzola | 1½ oz | 155 | Plaice, boiled | 6 oz | 84 |
| processed | 1½ oz | 135 | Prawns, boiled | 4 oz | 120 |
| Cream, single | 1 oz | 62 | Salmon, steamed | 4 oz | 216 |
| double | 1 oz | 131 | canned | 3 oz | 117 |
| Eggs, boiled | 1 (2 oz) | 92 | Sardines, solids | | |
| fried | 1 (2 oz) | 136 | and oils | 2 oz | 168 |
| Milk | 6 oz | 114 | solids only | 2 oz | 120 |
| condensed | ½ oz | 50 | Shrimps, boiled | 4 oz | 128 |
| dried, skimmed | 6 oz | 60 | Sole, steamed | 4 oz | 96 |
| evaporated | 1 oz | 41 | Tuna | 3 oz | 220 |
| Yoghurt (plain), | | | | | |
| low fat | 5 oz | 75 | **Beverages** | | |
| (flavoured) | 5 oz | 120 | Orange, lemon, | | |
| | | | grapefruit | | |
| **Meat and poultry** | | | squashes | 2 oz | 72/78 |
| Bacon | 2 oz | 360 | Bovril | 5 oz | 5 |
| Beef, roast | 2 oz | 218 | Chocolate, | | |
| (lean only) | 2 oz | 128 | drinking | 5 oz | 175 |
| stewed steak | 3 oz | 164 | Coca-cola | 11½ oz | 125 |
| corned beef | 3 oz | 198 | Coffee | 6 oz | 6 |
| Chicken, | | | Coffee (half milk, | | |
| boiled or roast | 4 oz | 216 | 2 tsp. sugar) | 5 oz | 115 |
| Duck, roast | 4 oz | 356 | Horlicks | ½ oz | 56 |
| Ham, boiled, lean | 2 oz | 124 | Lucozade | 6 oz | 114 |
| Heart | 3 oz | 81 | Ovaltine | ½ oz | 54 |
| Kidneys, stewed | 3 oz | 135 | Oxo | 1 cube | 15 |
| Lamb or mutton | | | Ribena | 2 oz | 130 |
| roast | 3 oz | 249 | Tea | 6 oz | 6 |
| chop, grilled | 3 oz | 324 | Tonic water | 11½ oz | 90 |
| Liver (ox), fried | 4 oz | 342 | | | |
| Pork, roast | 3 oz | 270 | **Alcohol** | | |
| chop, grilled | 3 oz | 276 | Beer | 1 pt | 160–220 |
| Sausages, beef | 3 oz | 243 | Cider | 10 oz | 110 |
| pork | 4 oz | 372 | Liqueurs | | 65–90 |
| Steak pie | 6 oz | 540 | Port | 2 oz | 86 |
| Tongue | 4 oz | 335 | Sherry, dry | 2 oz | 66 |
| Tripe | 4 oz | 115 | sweet | 2 oz | 76 |
| | | | Spirits | 1 oz | 63 |
| **Fish and shellfish** | | | Stout | 10 oz | 100 |
| Cod, steamed | 8 oz | 184 | Wines, white | 4 oz | 84–102 |
| fried | 8 oz | 464 | red | 4 oz | 72–80 |
| Fish fingers | 3 (3 oz) | 145 | | | |
| Haddock | 6 oz | 168 | | | |
| Herring, soused | 6 oz | 324 | | | |
| Mackerel, boiled | 6 oz | 234 | *Note: 1 oz = 30 grams approx.* | | |

# Cholesterol and saturated fats

| Fruit | Cholesterol | Saturated fats |
|---|---|---|
| Apples | nil | nil |
| Bananas | nil | nil |
| Grapefruit | nil | nil |
| Grapes | nil | nil |
| Melon | nil | nil |
| Oranges | nil | nil |
| Peaches, fresh | nil | nil |
| Pears, fresh | nil | nil |
| Pineapple, fresh | nil | nil |
| Raspberries | nil | nil |
| Raisins | nil | nil |

| Vegetables | Cholesterol | Saturated fats |
|---|---|---|
| Beans, all sorts | nil | nil |
| Brussels sprouts | nil | nil |
| Cabbage | nil | nil |
| Cauliflower | nil | nil |
| Celery | nil | nil |
| Lettuce | nil | nil |
| Mushrooms | nil | nil |
| Onions | nil | nil |
| Parsnips | nil | nil |
| Peas | nil | nil |
| Potato salad | high | high |
| Potatoes | nil | nil |
| Spinach | nil | nil |
| Tomatoes | nil | nil |
| Watercress | nil | nil |

| Nuts | Cholesterol | Saturated fats |
|---|---|---|
| Peanuts | nil | medium |
| Other nuts | nil | low |

| Cereals and cereal products | Cholesterol | Saturated fats |
|---|---|---|
| Bread, white or brown | nil | low |
| Cereals | nil | low |
| Water biscuits | nil | low |
| Spaghetti, macaroni, noodles | nil | low |
| Egg pastas | medium | medium |

| Oils and fats | Cholesterol | Saturated fats |
|---|---|---|
| Corn oil | nil | low |
| Lard, suet | medium | high |
| Peanut oil | nil | medium |
| Soya bean oil | nil | low |
| Sunflower oil | nil | low |
| Mayonnaise | medium | medium |
| Peanut butter | nil | low |

| Cakes and desserts | Cholesterol | Saturated fats |
|---|---|---|
| Cakes | high | high |
| Biscuits, sweet | low | medium |
| Ice cream | medium | high |
| Pancakes | medium | medium |

| Dairy products | Cholesterol | Saturated fats |
|---|---|---|
| Butter | medium | high |
| Margarine, soft | nil to medium | high |
| other | nil to medium | high |
| Cream | high | high |
| Cheese, whole milk | medium | high |
| skimmed milk | low | low |
| cottage | low | low |
| Egg, boiled | high | low |
| fried | high | medium |
| Egg white | nil | nil |
| yolk | high | low |
| Milk | medium | medium |
| evaporated | medium | high |
| skimmed | low | low |

| Meat and poultry | Cholesterol | Saturated fats |
|---|---|---|
| Beef | medium | high |
| Heart | high | medium |
| Kidney | high | low |
| Lamb | medium | high |
| Liver | high | low |
| Pork, bacon | medium | high |
| Sausages (fresh) | medium | high |
| Veal | medium | medium |
| Chicken | medium | low |
| Duck | medium | high |
| Turkey | medium | low |

| Fish and shellfish | Cholesterol | Saturated fats |
|---|---|---|
| Shrimps | high | low |
| Other shellfish | high | low |
| Roe | high | medium |
| Wet fish | medium | low |

# Metabolic costs

It is important that a patient suffering from coronary artery disease (or any other disorder) should know just what physical activity he is capable of, and precise instructions should be given relevant to his specific problem. Standard exercise testing procedures can usually provide information on an individual's potential activity if this is limited in any way, whether in relation to the heart or elsewhere.

The tables below show the approximate metabolic cost of different activities; to understand them certain terms must be clarified:

*1. METs (metabolic equivalents)*     This is a most useful unit of measurement – so far, more widely used in the United States than elsewhere – because it is not dependent on body weight. One MET is the energy required while sitting and awake. All other activities are expressed as multiples of this basic requirement: for example, getting dressed requires twice the amount of energy needed for sitting, i.e. 2 METs.

*2. Oxygen consumption*     Every activity requires a certain amount of oxygen uptake and utilization by the body. When this consumption is assessed as the amount of oxygen used per unit of body weight, it will usually be the same amount of oxygen for all individuals whatever the difference in total body weight – particularly if the activity involves body movement. The measurement is determined as millilitres of oxygen consumed per minute per kilogram of body weight: $O_2$ml/min/kg. Oxygen uptake is probably the best single indication of physical fitness.

*3. Calories*     The calorie is the older, more familiar unit of heat production or energy expenditure. Because of the significance of body weight in its use it is not now so commonly adopted. For all individuals, certain factors will increase the energy requirements for any activity:

*Personal factors*
  (a)  digestion of meals
  (b)  cigarette smoking
  (c)  poor loss of body heat through skin and sweating
  (d)  emotional stress

*Environmental factors*
   (a) extremes of temperature
   (b) high humidity
   (c) high altitude
   (d) increased wind velocity

*Other factors*
   (a) physical fitness and conditioning
   (b) nature of work (body position)
   (c) knack at the job (skill and coordination, rhythm, self-confidence)
   (d) frequency and duration of rest period

The following table gives a general classification for normal and industrial activities.

| Activity | METs |
|----------|------|
| Light | 1–2 |
| Moderate | 2–4 |
| Heavy | 4–6 |
| Very heavy | 6–8 |
| Unduly heavy | over 8 |

In order to ascertain the physical capabilities of a patient, it is necessary to have some guide related to his symptoms. The following was drawn up by the American Heart Association.

*Functional classification of patients with heart disease*

1. Patients with heart disease but without resulting limitation of physical activity: i.e. ordinary physical activity does not produce undue fatigue, palpitations, shortness of breath or angina.

2. Patients with heart disease resulting in slight limitation of physical activity: i.e. they are comfortable at rest but ordinary physical activity results in fatigue, palpitations, shortness of breath or angina.

3. Patients with cardiac disease resulting in marked limitation of physical activity: i.e. they are comfortable at rest but less than ordinary physical activity causes fatigue, palpitations, shortness of breath or angina.

4. Patients with cardiac disease resulting in inability to carry out any physical activity without discomfort: symptoms such as angina may be present at rest and any activity increases discomfort.

**Functional classification and MET equivalents**

| Met | 1 | 2 3 4 | 5 6 | 7 8 9 10 11 12 13 14 15 |
|---|---|---|---|---|
| Functional classification | **4** | **3** | **2** | **1** |

Using these classifications with the following tables it is possible to find out exactly what an individual's capabilities should be. It must be stressed that real physical fitness is achieved gradually and only maintained by continuing with regular exercise, preferably three times a week.

| METs 1½–2 | ml 0₂/min/kg 4–7 |
|---|---|

**METs 1½–2   ml O₂/min/kg 4–7**

*Domestic*
Conversation
Dressing
Eating
Hand sewing
Polishing furniture
Shaving
Standing (relaxed)
Sweeping floor
Wheelchair propulsion

*Occupational*
Armature winding
Bookbinding (light)
Car driving
Clerical work
Knitting
Power sanding or sawing
Watch repairing

*Recreational*
Flying
Knitting
Motorcycling
Painting (sitting)
Playing cards
Strolling (1 mph)

**METs 2–3   ml O₂/min/kg 7–11**

*Domestic*
Cleaning windows
Ironing (standing)
Kneading dough
Making beds
Peeling potatoes
Walking (2 mph)
Washing hands, face
Washing small clothes
Wiping floors (light, kneeling)

*Occupational*
Bartending
Car repairs
Janitorial work
Radio/TV repairs
Shoe repairs
Typing

*Recreational*
Billiards
Bowling
Canoeing (2½ mph)
Cycling on level (5 mph)
Fly fishing (land)
Horse riding (at walk)
Playing musical
    instrument
Playing with children (light)
Walking on level (2 mph)
Woodwork (light)

**METs**    **ml $0_2$/min/kg**
3–4        11–14

*Domestic*
Beating carpets
Cleaning windows
Hanging up washing
Mopping
Taking a shower (warm)
Wringing by hand

*Occupational*
Bricklaying
Machine assembly
Plastering
Ploughing (tractor)
Driving trailer in traffic
Welding (moderate load)
Wheelbarrow (100kg, 220lb, load)

*Recreational*
Archery
Badminton (social doubles)
Cycling (6 mph)
Fly fishing (wading, still water)
Gardening or weeding (light)
Horse riding (sitting to trot)
Pushing light power mower
Sailing (handling small boat)
Walking (2½ mph)

**METs**    **ml $0_2$/min/kg**
4–5        14–18

*Domestic*
Scrubbing floor (heavy, kneeling)
Stripping a bed
Walking (3–4 mph)
Walking downstairs

*Occupational*
Carpentry (light)
Ploughing (horse)
Paperhanging
Painting, masonry
Wheelbarrow (50kg, 110lb,
   at 2½ mph)

*Recreational*
Badminton (singles)
Cycling (8 mph)
Dancing (foxtrot, waltz)
Gardening (heavy)

Hoeing
Many calisthenics
Raking leaves
Swimming (light)
Table tennis
Tennis (doubles)
Walking (3–4 mph)

**METs**    **ml $0_2$/min/kg**
5–6        18–21

*Occupational*
Carpentry (heavy)
Digging garden
Sawing soft wood
Shovelling light earth

*Recreational*
Cycling (10 mph)
Gymnastics (hopping)
Horse riding (rising to trot)
Ice or roller skating
Sexual activity (marital)
Stream fishing (wading in light
   current)

**METs**    **ml $0_2$/min/kg**
6–7        21–25

*Occupational*
Binding sheaves
Shovelling (10kg, 22lb, in 10 mins)

*Recreational*
Badminton (competitive)
Cycling (11 mph)
Dancing (square, rumba)
Lawn mowing (hand)
Shovelling light snow
Splitting wood
Tennis (singles)
Walking (5 mph)

**METs**    **ml $0_2$/min/kg**
7–8        25–28

*Occupational*
Carrying 80kg, 175lb
Digging ditches, spading
Felling trees
Planing

Sawing hardwood
Shovelling heavy snow
Self help: ambulation (braces and
  crutches)

*Recreational*
Canoeing (4 mph)
Cycling (12 mph)
Horse riding (gallop)
Ice hockey
Jogging (5 mph)
Mountain climbing
Swimming (backstroke)

**METs**      **ml 0$_2$/min/kg**
  8–9          28–32

*Occupational*
Shovelling (14kg, 31lb, in 10 mins)
Tending furnace

*Recreational*
Cycling (13 mph)
Fencing
Running (5½ mph)
Squash (social)

**METs**      **ml 0$_2$/min/kg**
over 10       over 32

*Occupational*
Ascending stairs (54 per min)
Shovelling (16+kg, 35+lb, in
  10 mins)

*Recreational*
Ski touring (5+ mph, loose snow)
Squash (competitive)

*Note: Emotional factors may
significantly increase energy
requirements*

# Glossary

*Adrenergic receptors*   Receivers in the heart which affect heart rate.

*Anaemia*   A medical condition with many causes in which there is a fall in the number of circulating red blood cells.

*Aneurysm*   A 'blow-out' in a blood vessel or heart wall due to a weakness in its structure.

*Angina*   Pain in the chest with characteristic distribution, usually brought on by exercise and relieved by rest.

*Angiogram*   X-ray investigation in which the outline of the heart chambers is seen by means of injected dye.

*Anterior descending artery*   A large artery which passes down over the front of the heart.

*Aorta*   The huge artery which leaves the left ventricle.

*Anti-coagulants*   A group of drugs used to delay blood clotting.

*Asystole*   When all electrical activity of the heart ceases and the heart stops beating.

*Atherosclerosis*   The ageing process of the arterial tree, involving the laying down of deposits within the vessels and loss of elasticity.

*Atrio-ventricular node*   Part of the electrical system of the heart, transferring the impulse from the sino-atrial node to the Bundle of His.

*Atrium*   One of two chambers of the heart which collect blood for transference to the ventricle.

*Beta blockers*   A group of drugs widely used in the treatment of heart disease which act by blocking the adrenergic receptors (see above).

*Bradycardia*   Abnormally slow heart rate.

*Bundle of His*   Part of the electrical system of the heart which transfers the impulse from the atrio-ventricular node to the ventricles.

*Cardiac catheterization*   A procedure in which a catheter is fed into the heart to relay dye so that the chambers of the heart and coronary artery circulation can be X-rayed.

*Catheter*   A narrow-bore tube, used in cardiac investigation as above.

*Cholesterol*   Naturally produced fat not containing a fatty acid.

*Cineangiography*   A method of taking a film of the heart as it is X-rayed, usually during cardiac catheterization.

*Circumflex artery*   A major artery of the coronary circulation – a branch of the left main coronary artery.

*Collagen*   Tough connective tissue found widely in the body.

*Defibrillation*   The application of an electrical current to the chest to restart a heart that has stopped beating.

*Diabetes*   A disease in which the sugar metabolism of the body is impaired.

*Diastolic pressure*   The lower reading of a blood pressure.

*Diuretics*   A group of drugs used to remove excess fluid from the body.

*Drip*   A method by which fluids are given into a vein.

*Dynamic exercise*   *See* Isotonic exercise.

*Echo-cardiogram*   Investigation of the heart using sound waves.

*Ectopics*   Bizarre heart beats which arise from an abnormal focus.

*Electrocardiogram (ECG)*   A machine which records the electrical activity of the heart as seen from different sites.

*Emphysema*   A condition of over-inflation of the chest wall resulting in poor air entry.

*Endarterectomy*   A surgical procedure involving the removal of plaque from an artery wall.

*Enzymes*   Complex organic substances, the levels of some of which may rise or fall in a heart attack.

*Ergometer*   A work machine (the term is usually applied to a static bicycle).

*Fibrosis*   The development of excessive fibrous tissue.

*Haemoglobin*   The red constituent of red blood corpuscles which carries oxygen.

*Haemorrhage*   Loss of blood from any source.

*Hypertension*   Blood pressure which is raised above acceptable levels.

*Hypotension*   Low blood pressure.

*Hypoxia*   A condition in which there are low levels of oxygen within the blood.

*Inferior vena cava*   The large vein returning to the right side of the heart from the lower body.

*Ischaemic heart disease*   A condition in which the heart muscle does not receive enough oxygen to meet demands.

*Isometric exercise*   A form of exercise in which the muscle fibres remain the same length, e.g. weight-lifting.

*Isotonic (or dynamic) exercise*   A form of exercise in which the muscle fibres change length and heart output is increased, e.g. running and cycling.

*Lipids*   A group of fats found in the bloodstream.

*Lipoprotein*   A chemical which transports cholesterol in the bloodstream.

*Mitral valve*   A valve in the heart situated between the left atrium and left ventricle.

*Occlusion*   A blockage, in the context of coronary artery disease usually applying to either partial or complete blockage of a blood vessel.

*Ophthalmoscope*   A diagnostic aid for viewing the inside of the eye, particularly in relation to the condition of the blood vessels.

*Oscilloscope*   A television-type screen used in monitoring hearts.

*Pacemaker*   Natural (or artificial – temporary or permanent) centre which controls the heart beat.

*Percutaneous transluminal angioplasty*  A new technique for the treatment of blocked coronary arteries which involves crushing the plaque on the vessel wall.

*Plaque*  A patch of deposit situated within the blood vessel wall.

*Platelets*  The constituent of blood active in the formation of blood clots.

*Pulmonary artery*  A large vessel taking deoxygenated blood from the heart to the lungs.

*Radio-telemetry*  A method of transmitting the electrical activity of the heart and then converting it into an ECG wave.

*Saturated fats*  Animal fats which are solid at room temperature.

*Septum*  The dividing wall between the two chambers of the heart.

*Sino-atrial node*  The centre of nerve cells in the electrical circuit of the heart.

*Sinus of Valsalva*  A pocket above the aortic valve from where the coronary arteries originate.

*Sphygmomanometer*  A diagnostic aid for recording and measuring blood pressure.

*Superior vena cava*  The large vein draining the head and neck and returning deoxygenated blood to the heart.

*Systolic pressure*  The higher of the two readings recorded in measuring blood pressure.

*Tachycardia*  Abnormally fast heart beat.

*Thrombus*  A blood clot within a blood vessel.

*Tricuspid valve*  A valve with three cusps between the right atrium and right ventricle.

*Triglycerides*  Compounds of glycerol and fatty acids.

*Unsaturated fats*  Fats (from vegetables or fish) which are liquid at room temperature.

*Ventricles*  The large muscular chambers of the heart: the right pumps blood to the lungs, the left to the body.

*Xanthalasma*  Deposits around the eyes, frequently associated with raised blood cholesterol.

# Index